The authors present a book whose subject will surprise many people... Yoga not only permits the mother to give birth in the best conditions and to quickly regain her equilibrium afterwards, but also combats certain cases of sterility in both sexes. Therefore, new horizons open for the couple.
Auxipress, Brussels, Belgium

This book is a very interesting study on how to give birth to a healthy and happy child. **Well illustrated ...many women will find excellent advice in it.**
Le Meridionnal La France, Marseille, France

Two experts on yoga, Anjali Devi Anand and Sri Ananda, affirm that certain positions have the power to re-establish the physiological equilibrium. Thus, yoga teaches how to master one's body, one's breathing, and one's thoughts. **This book, especially conceived for pregnant women, will show you the steps to follow.**
Figaro Madame, Paris

By the same author
in
Orient Paperback
Yoga : Develop Your Latent Powers (*illus.*)
Complete Book of Yoga : Harmony of Body and Mind (*illus.*)

YOGA
For Easier Pregnancy
& Natural Childbirth

Anjali Devi Anand
Sri Ananda

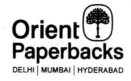
Orient Paperbacks
DELHI | MUMBAI | HYDERABAD

ACKNOWLEDGEMENTS

The authors wish to thank Swami Nityabodhananda of the Order of Sri Ramakrishna Paramahamsa, Madame M.A. Hameau, Mrs B. Abet-Luu-Van (M.D.), Dr E. Brunner and Dr W. Bubb for their interest and precious advice as regards the present work.

We would also like to thank the pupils at our Centre for agreeing to pose for the photographs contained in the present book.

www.orientpaperbacks.com

ISBN : 978-81-222-0240-3

1st Published 1988
This edition 2015

Yoga: For Easier Pregnancy & Natural Chidbirth
(Translated from the French by Alastair D. Panwell
with the help of the authors)

Asana photographs by Anjali Devi Anand,
teacher of *Hatha Yoga* at the Centre Indien de Yoga, Paris,
and Sri Ananda and their pupils

© Anjali Devi Anand and Sri Ananda

Cover design by Vision Studio

Published by
Orient Paperbacks
(A division of Vision Books Pvt. Ltd.)
5A/8 Ansari Road, New Delhi-110 002

Printed in India at
Ravindra Printing Press, Delhi-110 006

The present work is based on the *Vedas,* the *Ayurveda,* the *Garbha Upanishad* and *Hathayoga*

★ ★ ★

Revealed by Lord Shiva the science of Yoga has been taught in India from master to disciple since the beginning of history. It is with profound respect and infinite gratitude that we pay homage to the great ancient exponents of *Hathayoga,* such as *Matsyendra, Goraksa,* and *Svatmarama.*

Worship to Shiva

The Lord of the Universe &
Lord of the Cosmic Rhythm of Life

O Lord of Rhythm, O Lord of Time,
According to Your will divine,
After the night follows the day,
The moon in cycles goes her way.
Months and seasons come and go,
Bring heat and cold and rain, or snow.

O Lord of Rhythm, O Lord of Time,
According to Your will divine,
The soul must go through human birth
To gain experience upon this earth.

Coming from the astral plane,
The eternal soul is born again,
Till free forever from selfishness,
She leaves her sorrow for happiness.

Through service to humanity,
She grows in love and purity.
When her earthly state she can transcend,
Her cycle of rebirths comes to an end.

O Nataraja your praise I am singing.
Your Cosmic Dance all things pervading,
Destruction brings for new creation,
Your foot uplifted brings salvation.

Of all that is, You are the source,
You are the life-creating Force.
May all our lives be prosperous,
Love-filled and harmonious.

O Lord Shiva, O Lord Supreme,
May all be peaceful and serene.
In every form I worship You,
In humbleness I bow to You.

Anjali Devi Anand

Contents

*May the Almighty shower His blessings on
mothers all over the world*

The Joy of Childbirth

The birth of a child is generally considered a blessing and a source of great joy. It arouses extremely tender feelings in all those close to the child, and is accompanied by various rituals and ceremonies in the different countries of the world.

It is a perfectly natural instinct to have children. The love between the mother and the father helps create a happy family atmosphere and the child forges a closer link between the parents. The mother and father ensure that their sons and daughters receive proper care, and create the best conditions for their children's physical and mental development.

There can be no doubt, however, that in a large family, it is impossible to give each child everything he needs, and the mother's health is often impaired by too many pregnancies one after the other. This explains why, in developing countries where there are too many children, a policy designed to curb the birth rate has become a necessity. A massive population explosion can be dangerous in regions where poverty and malnutrition are endemic.

Most countries of the world have recognised the need to limit the number of births in accordance with each family's financial resources. The contraceptive methods developed over the past few years, which make it possible to keep the birth rate down, should not however prevent parents from having children or remove their responsibilities by ensuring that they do not produce any offspring. The industrialised countries indeed run the risk of a catastrophic drop in population, thereby creating a dangerous imbalance in the population of the world as a whole.

What counts most of all is to bring healthy, and well-balanced children into the world, capable of becoming men and women of great worth. The present modest work is intended to help parents achieve that aim and enable future mothers to enjoy perfect all-round health during pregnancy as well as to ensure that labour and delivery take place in the best possible conditions —thanks to the practice of *Hathayoga*.

Yoga and Hathayoga

Before proceeding to the actual practice of Hathayoga, we must know what it exactly means. The words *Ha* and *Tha* mean sun and moon. They refer to the vital currents circulating throughout our body. Solar energy—*prana*—is positive, while lunar energy—*apana*[1]—is negative. Hathayoga is the control and union of these two energies.

According to Swami Vivekananda, *Yoga* is the control of the senses, willpower and mind. To achieve this goal, one may begin by purifying oneself physically. Hathayoga is the system of Yoga specifically designed to allow for the purification of the body and mind. It is impossible, however, to achieve this by practising a series of physical exercises and nothing else. Unless the exercises are accompanied by the observance of mental discipline and certain moral rules, they will remain useless. Thus Hathayoga is also a way of life which enables those who practise it to lead a healthy, well-balanced and wise existence. Hathayoga consists of the following practices:

Pranayama: mastery of the body's vital forces through breath control,

The Kriyas: means of purification,

The Asanas: yogic postures,

The Mudras: seals and symbols and

The Bandhas: voluntary contractions of a group of muscles.

What does the term *Pranayama* mean? The word *Pranayama* is formed of *Prana* and *Ayama*. *Prana* is the omnipresent force manifesting itself in the universe. Everything which goes under the name of energy emanates from prana, which is also the vital force in each and every human being. *Ayama* means expansion and control of the vital forces.

Thus Pranayama is not breathing, as some have translated it, but a means of controlling the nerves and muscles related to breathing. It is the mastery of the muscular force moving the lungs. Thus it is the control of the lung

---

1. *Apana.* the specific name of the *prana* controlling the eliminatory functions of the body and the ejaculation of sperm.

movements associated with breathing—for according to Swami Vivekananda, "the most obvious manifestation of prana in the human body is the motion of the lungs".

There are six *Kriyas* or means of purification—*dhauti, basti, neti, nauli, kapalabhati* and *tratak*. These ensure the purification of the stomach, colon, nose, abdominal organs and lungs.

Tratak means fixing one's gaze without blinking on a point :

1) between the eyebrows called *Bhrumadhya-drishti,*
2) on the tip of the nose known as *Nasagra-drishti* and
3) on some other specific object. Although it is one of the Kriyas, it is specifically designed to stabilise and purify the mind, while at the same time developing the power of concentration.

There is also the *antar tratak,* which means directing one's attention within oneself, e.g., closing the eyes and keeping the consciousness on the space between the eyebrows i.e., seat of the third eye or on the heart centre—seat of the spiritual heart.

The asanas can be divided into two groups: meditation postures and physical postures.

The purpose of the physical postures is to produce a physiological balance between the different systems of the body—muscular, respiratory, circulatory, digestive, urinary, nervous and glandular system. The aim being to provide them with maximum organic vigour.

The asanas are usually practised for health reasons, but one should not forget that their ultimate purpose is, above all, the revitalisation of the spinal column, and through it and also through other parts of the body, to train the spinal chord and the brain, thereby preparing these for the awakening of the *Kundalini*[2], i.e. the spiritual energy which lies coiled and dormant at the base of the spinal column.

Advanced Yoga adepts practise the asanas, mudras, kriyas, bandhas and pranayama in order to control their sexual energy, for this is the only way of arousing the spiritual energy —i.e. *Kundalini Shakti.*

This advanced, esoteric practice of Hathayoga is strictly a monastic discipline—involving chastity and the renouncement of wordly things—which paves the way towards *Rajayoga* that leads one to the ultimate form of spiritual emancipation—*Kaivalya.*

Meditation postures allow a suitable position of the body for breathing exercises, bandhas, pranayama, tratak, concentration and, of course, meditation.

The mudras and bandhas are primarily concerned with the spiritual practice of Hathayoga, designed to arouse the Kundalini. On a physical level, their purpose is the control of the involuntary muscles and organs which are connected to the nerves and hence direct prana—vital energy—throughout the body. Certain of these mudras and bandhas, e.g. *Yogamudra* and *Uddiyana-*

2. cf. Sri Ananda, *Yoga—Harmony of Body and Mind,* Chapter I, Orient Paperbacks, Delhi; and Sri Ananda, *Yoga—Develop Your Latent Powers,* Chapter 2, Orient Paperbacks, Delhi.

Bandha, can be practised by everyone except on the occasions when they can be harmful. When performed correctly, the mudras and bandhas are extremely beneficial to ones's health.

The present work is devoted to the question of procreation and maternity. We have selected a series of exercises which primarily affect the nervous, glandular, circulatory and digestive systems. If these systems function properly, they can often remedy male impotence and sterility in both sexes.

In the chapter specifically written for pregnant women, we have chosen exercises which foster a normal pregnancy and lead to an anxiety-free childbirth with a minimum of discomfort.

Practised with patience and perseverance, Hathayoga is recommended to parents wishing to produce healthy children.

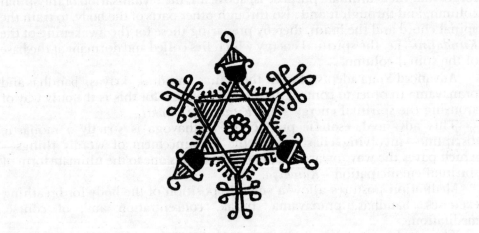

Sex During Pregnancy

Nature has endowed every living being with the need to reproduce. Sexual union between men and women should have no other natural purpose than procreation, i.e., to ensure the production of offspring. The mating of animals gives life to new beings, but in the case of man, physical union is not just a matter of conception, but also of pleasure. It is the excess of ·pleasure, however, which constitutes a perversion of this natural force.

The mating periods of animals are governed by natural laws and occur only at certain precise moments of the year. Once she has conceived, the female animal refuses sexual relations with the male. Unfortunately, human beings transgress this law, although it is very important to the health of parents and offspring alike. If parents do not observe certain rules, they run the risk of producing weak or sickly children.

A certain degree of continence or sexual control is therefore highly necessary, and even indispensable, to the health of the couple and for that of future generations, and can be achieved by practising Yoga.

Continence achieved through Yoga favours the regeneration of the reproductory cells, tissues and glands, and by revitalising the body it helps the individual· cope with life's problems. It also helps save physical and mental energy, fortifies the mind and memory, calms the nerves, and leads one to attain peace.

According to the law of nature, men and women should only unite to reproduce, and once conception has taken place, they should cease all sexual relations so that the future child is healthy and strong.

The same principle is found in the Ayurveda[1], a very ancient system of Hindu medicine which states that one should not overuse this creative·force and that a man should only have intercourse with his wife in between her menstrual periods, and only when both of them wish to produce a child.

---

1. *Ayurveda* : *Ayur* means life and *Veda* means science, i.e. science of life; it also means science of living.

In today's society, it seems extremely difficult to apply these rules, and for some people it is impossible. The Indian Yogis advocate moderation as the solution to the problem. A well-balanced sex life satisfies the needs of body and mind.

As regard to intercourse during pregnancy parents should refrain from having sexual relations, in the interest of their future child, from the sixth month of pregnancy.

Once the child is born, the mother needs at least six weeks of rest and abstinence from sex in order to recover her strength and to allow her organs to revitalize to their original state so that future pregnancies are without complications.

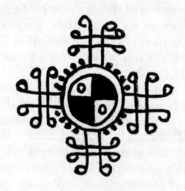

Yoga and Sterility

For many couples, the inability to have children is a great tragedy, for it seems unnatural and makes them feel frustrated. A man who does not have a son to carry on his name often feels disappointed and even bitter. A woman who has never given birth to a child and has never held her newborn baby in her arms may feel deprived of one of life's deepest emotional satisfactions and may feel jealous of women who are mothers. Often childless women feel guilty, and this can be a source of despair. In almost every age and country, barren women have been despised and rejected. Unfortunately, today, even in some countries, a man repudiates a wife who does not bear him any descendants. In many cases, it was thought that such women were being punished by the gods for their former sins, and the women in question were prepared to go to any lengths in order to produce a child. The entire blame for sterility was unjustly laid on them, whereas today we now know that it is the responsibility of the husband to see the doctor. If a couple has no children, both partners should consult a doctor in order to find out which of them requires treatment. Medicine has made solid progress in this field, e.g. a woman suffering from an inverted uterus can easily be cured. Likewise, fertilisation hampered by diseased ovaries or constricted Fallopian tubes can often be remedied.

A woman who has difficulty in conceiving would be well advised to consult a gynaecologist to find out the dates of the month most favourable for her to conceive.

As for the husband, he may perhaps due to seminal weakness not produce any or not enough spermotozoa or have blocked canals or have other problems which can be medically cured.

The doctor will suggest biological tests of the sperm, if it is the husband who is sterile, and will investigate the endocrine problems, if it is the wife.

According to Yoga, sterility can be either due to the couple's state of health, or also due to psychological factors. Malnutrition, serious disease, and poor living conditions will not of themselves stop fertility, but observation has revealed that men who are too tense or nervous are unable to produce the spermatozoon required for fertilisation. After proper rest and a suitable diet, these same men are able to have children. Similarly, it has been shown that the fear of being unable to conceive often prevents a woman from becoming pregnant. Couples who after years of sterility decide to adopt a child sometimes conceive one of their own a few months later, for once reassured, the wife is able to reproduce.

We may therefore conclude that in certain cases, sterility is caused by infinitely subtle psychological mechanisms. It is important not to overlook a suitable diet as a way of remedying sterility. Women who are extremely thin or anaemic are sometimes unable to conceive, but become pregnant the moment they gain weight and follow an adequate diet, rich in proteins, i.e. milk, cheese, dry vegetables, lentils, dhal, beans, peas, chickpeas, soyabeans, cereals, eggs, meat and fish. Overweight women have often produced a baby after dieting to lose weight.

The nervous system has a powerful effect on the glandular system, and nervous troubles can even lead to a deterioration in the endocrine glands which maintain the physiological balance of the human body.

A glandular system which functions poorly can be the root cause of premature ageing and genital problems which prevent reproduction in the case of both men and women. Thyroid problems can also be a cause of sterility.

The sexual glands produce not only genetic material, i.e. the cells needed for reproduction, but also chemical substances known as hormones which, among their other functions, have a revitalising effect on the body. Thus it is essential for them to be in good working order. Intermittent impotence, lack of libido, loss of virility and frigidity can produce a negative effect on a couple's harmony.

16

Asanas Favourable For Conception

The regular and conscientious practice of Hathayoga allows one to keep fit by preserving and expanding one's physical and mental faculties. It slows down the ageing process and helps one remain strong and active, well upto old age.

Warning

The exercises indicated in the present book can be harmful if they are performed incorrectly and without the guidance of a qualified instructor. Before accepting a pupil, the teacher should be informed about the pupil's state of health and he should offer the pupil necessary advice on how to carry out the exercises correctly.

Some exercises should not be performed by menstruating women; by those suffering from spinal problems or with hyper or hypotension, and with various other problems such as asthmatic and heart problem or orthopaedic ailmens like arthritis, ostoarthritis, muscle spasms etc. The exercises in question can be modified or replaced with more suitable yogic practices.

The exercises must not be practised during digestion period. They should be performed before eating, or at least 4½ hours after a substantial meal.

Obviously, a choice must be made from the exercises described in the present chapter. These should be practised during a complete session of Hathayoga. The asanas marked with an asterisk (*) should not be performed during menstruation.

The duration and number of repetitions for each exercise should gradually be increased, in strict accordance with the instructor's guidance. At the end of a Yoga session, one should not feel tired, but exact the opposite, i.e. fresh and full of energy.

The following are the asanas, including one mudra and one bandha, which are recommended for fostering reproduction and combatting impotence and sterility. Some of the postures reappear in either modified or original form in the chapters devoted to 'For Easier Childbirth and a Healthy Baby: Asanas and Exercises During Pregnancy[1].'

---

1. For the technique used in the following exercises, see Sri Ananda's book *Yoga—Harmony of Body and Mind,* Orient Paperbacks Delhi.

Asanas

The Yogic Postures

Sirshasana* : The Head-stand

All human activity, whether mental or physical, is governed by the brain, and the nervous system is directly linked to this organ.

By performing *Sirshasana* or the head-stand, one causes an abundant influx of arterial blood to the brain, thereby 'irrigating' and regenerating not only this organ but the entire nervous system.

Some of the most important endocrine glands, situated in the area above the heart—hypophysis, pineal and thyroid, but particularly the first two—are regenerated and maintained in perfect health by the head-stand.

The digestive and excretory organs will also function better in cases where their malfunctioning is due to a poor circulation, the descent of organs or a generally deficient nervous system. This posture helps combat psycho-somatic imbalance and ensures that the organs remain highly active.

It has beneficial effects in cases of hernia and constipation. It also provides a remedy for seminal weakness. Since the testicles are situated between the bladder and the rectum, if these become overfull, especially the rectum of people who are constipated, nocturnal emissions may take place. The head-stand is extremely effective as far as this problem is concerned.

Sirshasana also helps prevent premature ejaculation, where this is caused by congestion of the genital organs. It is also excellent for women suffering from certain uterine or ovarian troubles, or from the downward displacement of the womb.

When practising Sirshasana, begin by remaining in this posture for five seconds, then gradually increase the length of time by fifteen seconds every week until a maximum of three minutes is reached. Be sure to practise this posture every day.

This asana should under no circumstances be performed by those with hyper or hypotension, weak cervical vertebrae, and also by those who are suffering from a heavy cold or have problems with their ears or eyes. Those with a weak heart should practise this posture with great care, and on no account should it be performed less than 30 minutes after strenuous exercise.

---

* All asanas marked with an asterisk (*) should not be performed during menstruation.

Sirshasana*

The Head-stand

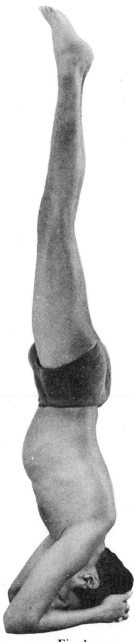

Fig. 1

Sarvangasana*

The Shoulder-stand

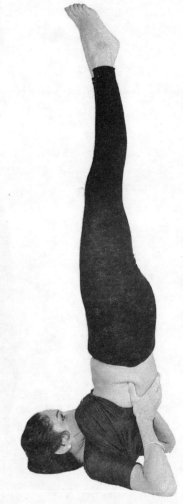

Sarvangasana* : The Shoulder-stand
This posture differs from Sirshasana, in that the head and neck are in a different position. The pressing of the chin against the hollow area situated above the sternum allows this asana to produce a more powerful effect on the thyroid gland.

Like Sirshasana, it remedies seminal weakness in men, arising from the degeneration of the testes, and gives a beneficial effect on the uterus and ovaries in women. It also ensures the correct functioning of the reproductory glands in both sexes.

Sarvangasana is the ideal posture for combatting female barrenness. It is also recommended for those suffering from ptosis or downward displacement of the womb.

Fig. 2

Sarvangasana is the asana *par excellence* for counteracting the faulty functioning of the thyroid and parathyroid glands, and for revitalising them. Situated in the neck region, these glands play a part in the correct functioning of the metabolism, influence one's state of mind, and produce a considerable effect on the sexual maturing process. This posture enables one to remain active to a great age.

The restrictions which apply to Sirshasana also apply to Sarvangasana. The exercise can be repeated once or twice in succession for fifteen seconds to three minutes. The duration must be increased gradually.

20

Matsyasana

The Fish Posture

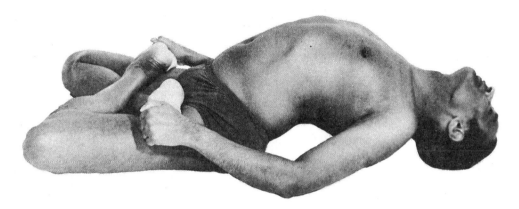

Fig. 3

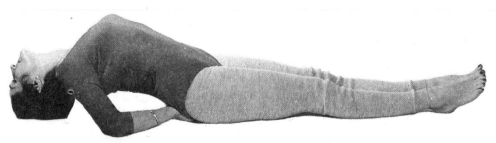

Fig. 4

Matsyasana : The Fish Posture (See technique p. 101)
This posture completes the preceding one i.e. Sarvangasana. It should be done for five seconds to one minute (i.e., one third of the time spent in Sarvangasana). This asana is usually performed once. It greatly helps the correct functioning of the thyroid gland (producing a tonic effect on it) and the endocrine system. It also eases constipation and in the case of women, ensures a healthy uterus.

21

Viparita Karani
The Inverted Position

Viparita Karani : The Inverted Position

This inverted posture revitalises the entire organism. It is easier to perform than the Sirshasana and the Sarvangasana. It combines the effects of both—Sirshasana and Sarvangasana, though less powerfully. *Viparita Karani* can be practised to replace both of them.

Viparita Karani can be practised one or two times in succession, lasting for fifteen seconds to three minutes—the duration should be increased gradually. It should not be performed by those suffering from high blood pressure.

Sirshasana, Sarvangasana and Viparita Karani are inverted positions which have a direct action on the brain, the thyroid and other endocrine glands. This action prevents premature ageing and rejuvenates the cells. These yogic postures are among the most important as far as fostering procreation is concerned.

The following asanas produce a far-reaching action on the pelvic and sacro-lumbar regions, as well as on the abdominal organs. They improve the circulation, thereby producing a tonic effect on the nerves connected to the sexual organs, and on the male and female reproductory glands. These asanas can therefore provide a remedy, in certain cases, for impotence and sterility.

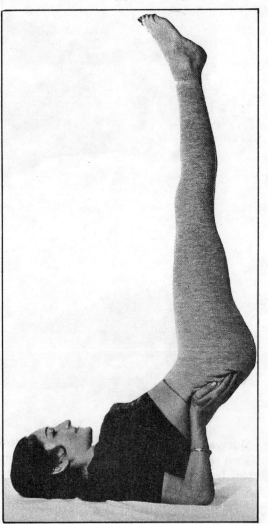

Fig. 5

Halasana*
The Plough Posture

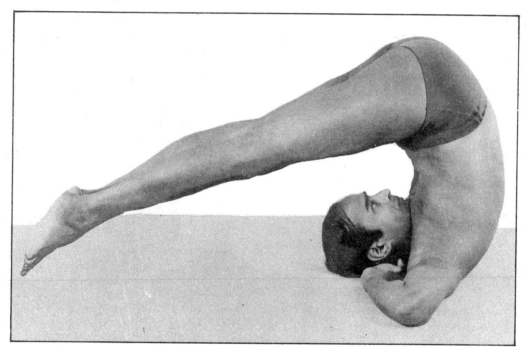

Fig. 6

Halasana* : The Plough Posture

This posture tones up the nerves of the spine linked to the sexual organs and the neuro-muscular system of the pelvic region. It combats dyspepsia and constipation, and has a beneficial effect on the liver. *Halasana* also regenerates the thyroid gland—in the third stage of this posture, the chin presses against the hollow region at the top of the sternum. (See Fig. 2).

In addition, this asana strengthens the male and female reproductory glands. It can be practised two or three times in succession for the duration of five seconds to one minute.

Bhujangasana
The Cobra Posture

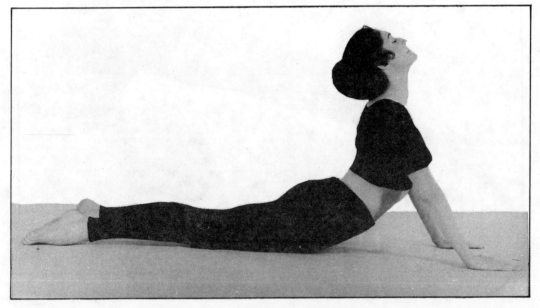

Fig. 7

Bhujangasana : The Cobra Posture

This posture helps the blood circulation, regenerates the spinal nerves, the sympathetic nervous system, and remedies insomnia. It combats flatulence and digestive problems, and, in the case of women, ensures a healthy uterus and ovaries. This asana also helps correct irregular menstruation.

Bhujangasana is performed two to five times over a period of five to ten seconds.

24

Dhanurasana
The Bow Posture

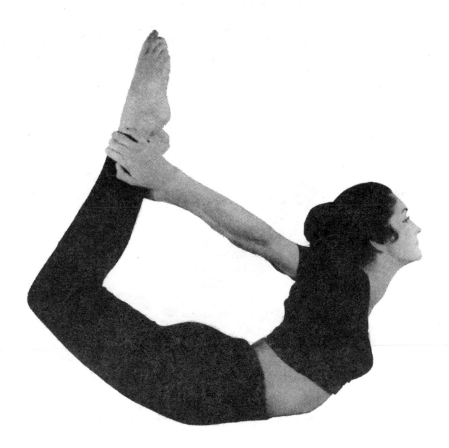

Fig. 8

Dhanurasana : The Bow Posture

This posture helps exercise the spinal column, the abdominal muscles and the articulation of the hips. It produces a tonic effect on the pelvic region and the digestive organs. It helps regenerate the male prostate gland, and the endocrine glands and genital organs of both sexes. It is also recommended to women as a way of ensuring proper functioning of uterus and ovaries. *Dhanurasana* can be performed two to five times for five seconds.

Salabhasana* and Ardha-Salabhasana
The Locust Posture and The Half-Locust Posture

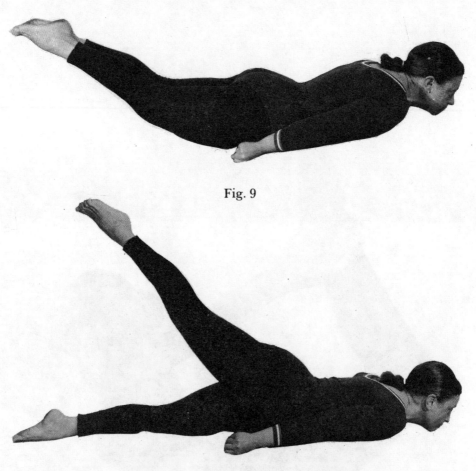

Fig. 9

Fig. 10

Salabhasana*and Ardha-Salabhasana   : The Locust Posture and the Half-Locust Posture

These two postures have an invigorating effect on the pelvic and abdominal regions, and on the male and female sexual organs. They produce a beneficial action on the urogenital system, the stomach and the intestines. *Salabhasana* and *Ardha-Salabhasana* ensure, in women, correct functioning of the ovaries and that menstruation is regular and painless. They should be practised two to five times in succession for several seconds.

The Cobra, Locust, Half-Locust and Bow postures are an excellent means of combatting female sterility resulting from the poor functioning of the reproductive organs and irregular menstruation.

26

Paschimottanasana*
The Posterior Stretching Posture

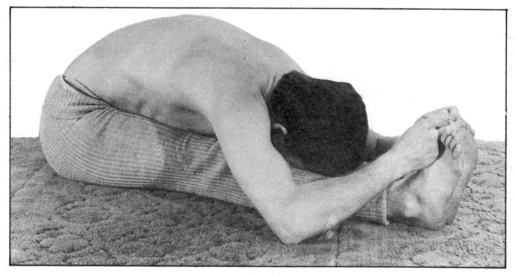

Fig. 11

Paschimottanasana* : The Posterior Stretching Posture
This posture is good for the sciatic nerve and especially beneficial to the sacro-lumbar, pelvic and abdominal regions, in which it tones up the blood circulation. It is an useful way of combatting constipation and dyspepsia. It revitalises the nerves connected to the genital organs as well as the sexual glands of both sexes. This asana is known·in India for its tonic effect on the organism as a whole and for remedying impotence. It is recommended as a way of curing seminal weakness and controlling sexual energy. *Paschimottanasana* is performed two to five times for five to ten seconds.

Janusirasana*
The Knee-and-Head Posture

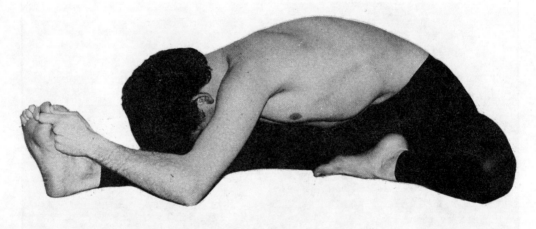

Fig. 12

Janusirasana* : The Knee-and-Head Posture
This posture is beneficial to the nerves of the spinal column which are linked to the genital organs. It is also good for the sciatic nerve, and the sacro-lumbar and pelvic regions. In addition, this asana promotes health to the prostate gland and helps cure prostatic enlargement problems. It also stimulates the abdominal organs.

In the case of women, this posture strengthens the uterine muscles and Fallopian tubes, while at the same time improving the functioning of the ovaries.

Janusirasana should be repeated two or three times on either side for five seconds.

28

Supta-Vajrasana
The Supine Pelvic Posture

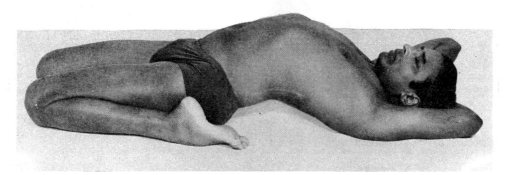

Fig. 13

Supta-Vajrasana : The Supine Pelvic Posture
This posture produces a highly revitalising effect on the reproductive organs and the entire pelvic region. It is also a powerful means of fighting constipation. The asana is performed two times in succession for fifteen to thirty seconds.

Ardha-Matsyendrasana

The Half-Matsyendra Posture

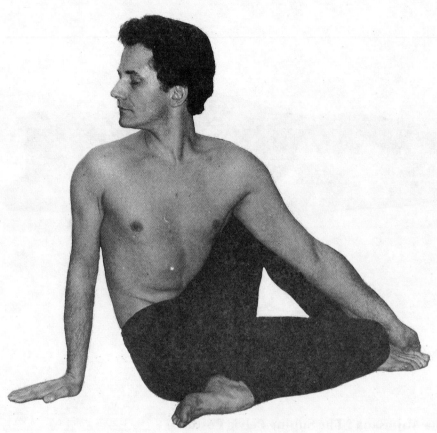

Fig. 14

Ardha-Matsyendrasana : The Half-Matsyendra Posture

This posture is effective against constipation and dyspepsia. It is very effective against an enlarged and congested liver and spleen, and revitalises the functioning of the kidneys, bladder and genital organs.

It guards against enlargement of the prostate gland, and continues to rejuvenate the spinal column and reproductive organs until quite late in life. When combined with some other postures, the tonic effects of this asana is increased.

Ardha-Matsyendrasana should be performed two or three times in succession for five to fifteen seconds on either side.

30

Badha-Konasana*

The Yoga-Mudra Feet Joined

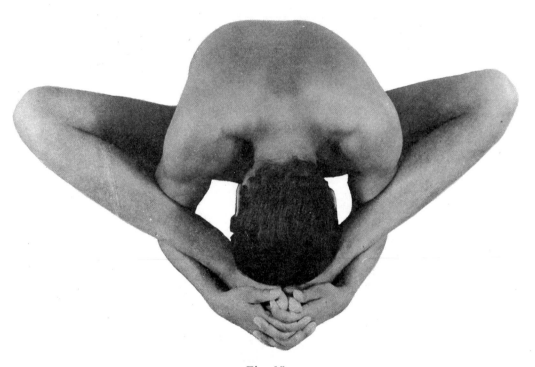

Fig. 15

Badha-Konasana* : The Yoga-Mudra Feet Joined
This posture stimulates the abdominal organs and the sacro-lumbar region, and ensures the correct functioning of the sexual organs. It helps ensure regular menstruation, and is recommended to those suffering from urinary problems.

Badha-Konasana should be repeated two or three times in succession for five to ten seconds.

31

Yoga-Mudra *
The Symbol of Yoga

Yoga-Mudra* : The Symbol of Yoga

This exercise stimulates the brain by provoking an influx of fresh blood. It has a rejuvenating effect on the coccygeal (i.e. tail-end of spinal column) nerves and on the sacral and lumbar plexus. It ensures the correct functioning of the abdominal organs and combats constipation. This asana also revitalises the male and female genital organs.

This Mudra remedies nocturnal emissions and seminal weakness. It also fosters control of sexual energy. *Yogamudra* plays a vital part in the spiritual (esoteric) practice of Hathayoga.

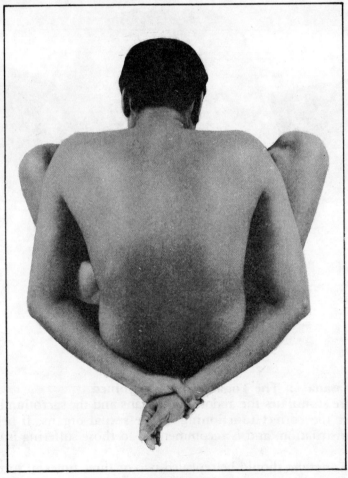

Fig. 16   Top-View

Uddiyana-Bandha[*]
The Raising of the Diaphragm

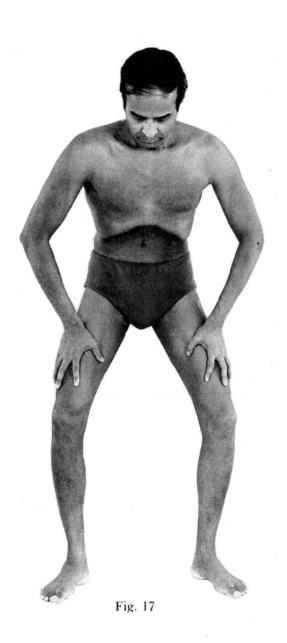

Fig. 17

Uddiyana-Bandha*: The Raising of the Diaphragm (See technique p. 142)

Uddiyana means 'raising up' and *Bandha* means 'voluntary contraction of a group of muscles.' This Bandha helps purify the organism, stimulate the digestive organs, and fight against constipation and dyspepsia. It ensures proper functioning of the liver, pancreas, suprarenal glands and genital organs.

This exercise revitalises the sacral and solar (lumbar) plexus—the latter of which controls the principal internal organs. The solar plexus is a vital centre connected with the sympathetic nervous system, a fact which explains why it also plays such an important part in the control of our emotions. It is the place where our vital energy—Prana is stored.

As its name suggests, the plexus in question is the sun of our nervous system. When functioning properly, it radiates strength and energy throughout the body.

Uddiyana-Banda is of great importance to the spiritual practice of Hathayoga. It should always be performed on an empty stomach, and is not recommended to those with high or low blood pressure or with serious problems affecting the blood circulation or the abdominal region. This Bandha may be repeated two to five times for five seconds.

As may be seen, the Asanas, the Mudra and the Bandha we have selected for the present chapter revitalise the sexual glands and organs, the thyroid, the nerves, and other organs which play an important part in reproduction.

We must emphasize, however, that one cannot expect the body and reproductive organs to function correctly if one overworks, smokes, drinks too much tea, coffee or alcohol, takes drugs, fails to eat a balanced diet, or indulges in emotional or sexual excess.

It is a well-known fact that the emotions exercise a considerable influence over the nervous system and the endocrine glands, and, by extension, the entire organism. Excessive emotion or passion is harmful, as we shall see in the following chapter.

Exercises For Overcoming Emotional Stress

I t is important to remember that the body and the mind are intimately linked. The influence of mind over body is, however, considerably greater than that of body over mind. It is the emotional aspect of mental activity which exercises the most powerful influence over the body—in particular, the nervous and endocrine systems.

A distinction must be drawn between positive emotions e.g., confidence, hope, joy, gratitude, devotion, etc., and negative ones e.g., rage, jealousy, despondency, fear, distress, envy, hatred, etc.

The positive emotions produce a generally beneficial effect on the nervous system, while the negative ones disrupt it. The endocrine system is thrown out of gear by negative emotions and this leads to illnesses which are sometimes quite serious, depending on the intensity and duration of the emotions in question.

The thyroid and sexual glands occupy an extremely important position among the endocrine glands. The sexual glands are very easily influenced by the emotions. For example, there have been cases where a violent emotional shock has caused sudden menstruation in women, or impotence in men. This is why it is important for us to learn to control our emotions and dominate over our impulses.

With this in mind, we recommend five highly useful exercises based on Savasana—complete yogic relaxation; Anuloma Viloma—breathing through alternate nostrils, rythmic breathing with autosuggestion; interiorisation and meditation.

Exercise 1

Savasana : Complete Yogic Relaxation Posture (See technique p. 103)
Lie on the back, and relax the different parts of the body one after the other until all tension disappears. For example, if someone lifts an arm, it should fall back as if completely inert. While relaxing, one should leave aside the problems of the outside world and everyday life.

A particular feature of this posture is that one is completely able, without actually dozing off, to detach oneself from the surrounding environment and to remain aware of one's deep physical and mental relaxation. In order to achieve this, regular breathing is required.

Persistent practice is needed to master this exercise (which is not at all easy to begin with) and to attain correct co-ordination between the relaxation of mind and body.

A perfectly relaxed psychosomatic system is one of the best remedies against anxiety and all forms of nervous or emotional tension.

Exercise 2
Anuloma Viloma : Breathing Through Alternate Nostrils
Like all the *Pranayama* exercises, this breathing technique generally includes a period of inhalation, *Puraka*, a period of retention, *Kumbhaka*, and a period of exhalation, *Rechaka*.

To begin with, the time spent on inhalation is half that of retention and exhalation, e.g. four seconds of inhalation, followed by eight seconds of retention and eight seconds of exhalation.

According to Swami Vivekananda, there are three kinds of Pranayama exercises: simple, intermediate and advanced. The second and third are not at all easy, and are only practised in India by monks who observe highly strict rules regarding their diet and their physical, moral and spiritual discipline. Without these rules, the exercises in question are not only useless but dangerous because they involve extremely long breathing periods and even longer retention periods. This can permanently damage the heart, nerves and lungs, especially if the lungs are not first strengthened and purified of all dust, smoke or other city pollution.

In the words of Swami[1] Kuvalayananda, a Yoga master and medical practitioner, those who practise Yoga uniquely for health reasons should not perform the retention of breath, for in this instance it serves no purpose.

According to Swami Kuvalayananda's laboratory experiments, it is not certain whether a larger quantity of oxygen is absorbed during the retention of the breath. On the other hand, the rate of four seconds inhalation and eight seconds exhalation which we recommend in the present chapter is the one most suitable for completely oxygenating the body.

The form of *Anuloma Viloma* which we therefore recommend does not involve retention of the breath. It is performed in a meditation posture, or sitting with the legs crossed. (See technique p. 109)

This exercise is to be performed three times a day--morning, noon and evening—before meals and can be repeated up to seven times in a session. During the first week, one should begin with three respirations per session; the second week, the number can be increased to five; thereafter, providing one performs the exercise every day, the number can reach a total of seven respirations—(actually 14 respirations through alternate nostrils.)

If practised regularly, Anuloma Viloma is one of the best exercises for

---

1. Swami—a Hindu monk belonging to an order.

purifying the nervous system and bringing calm to the mind. It is particularly recommended to those suffering from anxiety or depression.

All Pranayama exercises regulate the secretion of hormones, revitalise the nervous system, oxygenate the body and ensure the correct functioning of the entire organism. They not only calm the emotions, but also remedy the physical damage caused by them. In addition, they help control sensory and mental activity.

Exercise 3
Rhythmic Breathing With Autosuggestion
This exercise is performed with the back upright, sitting either in a meditation posture or cross-legged. Close the eyes and perform complete yogic breathing, i.e. abdominal, middle-chest and upper-chest or clavicular.

Breathe deeply and consciously, ensuring that the breathing rhythm respects an equal time for inhalation as for exhalation. Instead of simply using numerals to count i.e., one, two, three, four, five...., regulate the breathing with the help of words suggesting positive things e.g. 'calm and peace'. Repeat them to yourself rhythmically and harmoniously during inhalation and exhalation so that, in the end, you identify with them.

Whenever we breathe in and out, we should think of peace, for in concentrating on it, we attain perfect joy and inner peace.

"The body is what the mind makes of it. It is but the outer covering of the mind, and is obliged to carry out whatever the mind tells it to do."

SWAMI VIVEKANANDA

Interiorisation
Directing One's Attention Inwardly

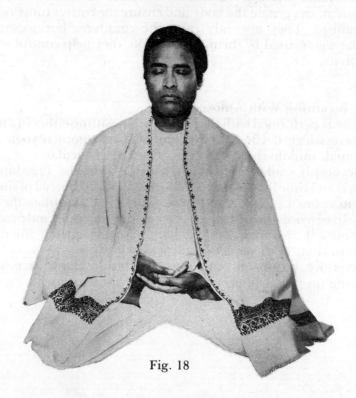

Fig. 18

Exercise 4
Interiorisation : Directing One's Attention Inwardly
In order to perform this exercise, assume a meditation posture, i.e. the Lotus, Half-Lotus or cross-legged position, with the back of the right hand resting in the palm of the left one.

Begin by regulating the breathing—a vital factor in stabilising the mind. After withdrawing from the outside world, allow the attention to remain centred on the depths of one's inner being while letting the mind bask in silence, calm and serenity. By collecting one's thoughts in this way, one is able to calm the baser instincts, dominate the impulses, and find inner harmony. Interiorisation and meditation are a unique therapy for psychosomatic illnesses. They help soothe the mind, produce a beneficial effect on the entire organism and revivify the nervous system.

Exercise 5
Meditation : Dhyana
A certain amount of preparation is required if meditation is to produce results. We advise those wishing to practise it to begin with the exercises described above. Once these have been performed regularly, one may then pass on to mediation.

38

Meditation
Dhyana

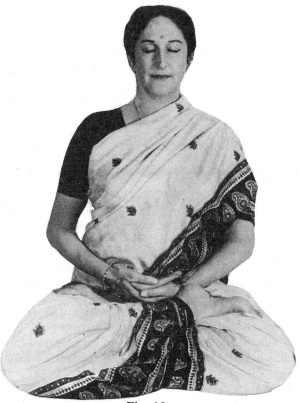

Fig. 19

Assume the same position as for interiorisation. Begin breathing rhythmically, for controlled breathing helps concentrate the mind and provides effective preparation for meditation.

Once a regular breathing pattern has been established, direct the attention towards the spiritual heart, located slightly to the right of the physical one. It is here, at the very core of our inner being, that the higher Self resides. It is the Soul of our soul, the Essence of our being, the Source of life within us.

While meditating on the Self, we are detached from material constraints, we go beyond the limitations of the body, and we transcend our awareness of the ego. This brings us great mental tranquillity and unfailing inner force; for human weaknesses stem from the fact that we constantly identify ourselves with the lower self which is limited and self-centred. By meditating on the supreme Self, as an unlimited and inexhaustible Force, we assert our will.

"The stronger the will, the less the yielding to the sway of the emotions."

SWAMI VIVEKANANDA

On Conceiving the Child

"Pure love, which is without claims or agressiveness, which does not seek to possess but to create a feeling of harmony, is the source of all bliss".

SWAMI NITYABODHANANDA

The sex drive is a natural instinct which prompts living beings to unite and reproduce. Intercourse should not, however, be based solely on mutual sexual satisfaction, but on the love shared by two people who bring to the sexual act all the tenderness and understanding required for its full consummation.

Parents who are aware of their responsibilities and who wish to produce a child possessing fine physical and moral virtues should avoid intercourse when they are tired, downcast or anxious, for their physical and mental state can affect the embryo from the moment it is conceived. For example, sexual acts under duress, rape or drunkenness at the moment of conception can cause physical damage to the future child. If all children were 'wanted', i.e. conceived in the best conditions and not as the result of an 'accident', mankind would be very different from what it is.

Indian sacred Scriptures state that intercourse should take place in a pleasant, harmonious atmosphere. The room used had to be clean, tidy, and decorated with religious images and pictures of fine landscapes. The belief was that if the parents were surrounded by beautiful things during the sexual act, their child would be attractive and healthy.

In the *Vedanta*, an extremely ancient holy text, emphasis is laid on the fact that between the 5th and the 11th day after her menstrual period, a woman should have nothing but positive, lofty thoughts. The reason for this is that these are the days most favourable to procreation, and with her emotions and thoughts the woman can profoundly affect her future child. The same text states that children conceived on the 6th, 8th, 10th, 12th, 14th or 16th day after menstruation (i.e. on the even days) will be boys, while those conceived on the odd days i.e., the 5th, 7th, 9th, 11th, 13th or 15th will be girls. It was noted that the woman who, at the moment of conception, breathed through her right nostril produced a son, while a woman who breathed through her left nostril gave birth to a daughter.

In Yoga, the right nostril is called *surya nadi, surya* meaning sun, while the left one is called *chandra nadi, chandra* meaning moon.

In his work *Ayurveda, the Science of Life,* Dr. C.G. Thakkur writes that if three or four drops of drugs such as Lakshmana or Sahadevi mixed with milk are poured into a woman's right nostril following impregnation, she may conceive a male child.

Present-day medical research in France and Canada seems to confirm that by following a suitable diet, a woman has an 80% chance of deciding the sex of her child. The future mother who wishes to have a boy should eat highly salted food which is rich in potassium. The woman wanting a girl should eat food with a high magnesium and calcium content for at least three and half months before conceiving the child.

Indian scriptures refer to prana—vital energy—which is also called the 'life-creating force'. The unification of the prana contained in the male sperm and the female ovule governs the development of the embryo in accordance with the law of *karma*[1]— the law of action and reaction forging one's destiny. Depending on the preponderance of either one or the other, the child will be a boy or a girl.

According to the *Garbha Upanishad*[2], written several thousand years ago, the child's body gradually develops inside the mother's womb. The text reads as follows:

"The first day after conception, the embryo looks like a nodule; seven days after, like a bubble; fifteen days later like a mass which hardens after one month.

"The head appears after two, i.e., lunar months, and part of the feet by the end of the third month. During the fourth month, the ankles, stomach and hips are formed, while during the fifth, the spinal column is formed, followed during the sixth month by the nose, eyes and ears. In the course of the seventh month, the embryo is equipped with a soul, *jiva,* and the child is completely formed by the eighth month."

Again according to the *Garbha Upanishad,* as of the ninth lunar month, the soul is able to remember her previous incarnations and actions, and knows why, depending on her karma, she must be reincarnated, i.e. be re-born. At the moment of birth, the soul is no longer able to remember her past, but in accordance with the law of *karma,* which is even and just, the individual will be drawn from his earliest childhood to situations and conditions of life which he will have deserved as a result of his thoughts and actions in former lives, and which will enable him to pass through the experiences necessary to his evolution.

The human soul, *jivatman,* must be incarnated in new physical bodies until she reaches Awareness, becomes free from all egoism and is filled with

---

1. *Karma :* law of cause and effect, of sowing and reaping.
2. Esoteric doctrine concerning the embryo.

universal Love. Only then will she achieve union with the supreme Soul, i.e., *Paramatman* and be released from the cycle of re-births. This is the ultimate goal of all systems of Yoga.

"Man is born a child. His power is the power to grow"

TAGORE

"In youth we should prepare for a happy old-age, and in old-age we should prepare for a happy life in the beyond."

MAHABHARATA

Important Tips For Pregnant Mothers

The first sign of pregnancy is the fact that menstruation comes to a halt. A woman who is pregnant generally experiences a feeling of weariness, inertia and irritability.

As early as the end of the first month, i.e: from four to six weeks after her last menstrual period, a woman can know for certain whether she is pregnant by undergoing a pregnancy test. This should be followed by a medical examination. Once she knows, she can follow the Yoga course specially reserved for pregnant women.

Expectant mothers sometimes suffer from morning-sickness. This can in many cases be avoided by eating some food in bed before getting up. Sometimes, pregnant women cannot abide certain smells or may salivate far more than usual. They may experience fits of giddiness or feel extremely tired. This is often due to lack of proteins, vitamins and minerals (iron in particular), a situation which can be rectified by means of an appropriate diet.

The mother-to-be will also find that her breasts grow heavier, while the nipples become larger and darker. Her bosom will expand and enlarge, and the volume of the uterus will increase. During pregnancy, a woman usually gains some ten to twelve kilos. All these changes are only temporary and should not be cause for alarm. A pregnant woman should say to herself that these symptoms are perfectly natural and accept them as they are.

Pregnant women should not smoke or drink. To avoid a miscarriage they should take care of themselves, avoid strenuous physical effort, and make sure not to carry or move objects that are too heavy. Long journeys(especially by car) and sports (other than walking and swimming) are not advisable.

The mother-to-be should pay attention to what she eats and avoid food that is heavy or difficult to digest. During the night, if she experiences cramps in the calves or toes, she should massage the affected parts and walk a few steps. A five to ten-minute footbath before the evening meal would provide relaxation to swollen ankles. Make sure the water is lukewarm and covers the calves, and add one soupspoon of sea salt per litre of water.

By the fourth month, the body has usually become accustomed to the hormonal change, and the future mother's psychic balance has been re-established. Unless it is her first pregnancy, she can feel the child moving inside her by the end of the sixteenth week.

During the fifth month, all pregnant women feel the baby moving. As for the baby, it begins to hear external noises, e.g. its parents' voices. At this stage in their development, many babies react when they hear certain sounds or when their surroundings are too quiet.

The future mother should begin paying special attention to the exercises which help avoid pains in the spinal column and lumbar region, fight against constipation, and improve the circulation.

During the sixth month, the baby's muscles grow stronger. The child begins to move more and turn around. Meanwhile the mother's legs begin to feel heavier, and she should practise yogic relaxation by raising them in a very precise manner in order to avoid blocking the circulation of the blood (See Fig 72). The pregnant woman shold avoid wearing high-feels or shoes which pinch the feet. She should also take food having enough iron and calcium, and it is imperative for her to see her doctor and dentist.

During the seventh month, the mother-to-be should make sure that she bends her knees and avoids twisting her spinal column when she wishes to pick up an object; and she should never carry items weighing more than ten kilos. She should relax, avoid tiring herself out, refrain from going on long journeys, especially by car, and make sure she gets enough sleep in order to avoid the kind of premature birth which occurs in women who are overtired.

During the eighth month, the mother's heartbeat is faster. She breathes more rapidly owing to an increased need for oxygen. Pressure on the bladder grows heavier, giving rise to a greater need to urinate. Some women find that most of the time they do not sleep well and experience pains in the groin and pubic region. In the West, doctors state that sexual relations should cease by the end of the 32nd week at the latest, i.e. the eigth lunar month. In India, couples are advised to refrain from intercourse much earlier.

During the ninth month, the oil massages of the bosom and stomach, begun during the third month, should be continued, for they help prevent stretch marks.

Generally speaking, during a woman's first pregnancy, the uterus rises extremely high at the end of the 36th week, thereby hampering abdominal (diaphragm) breathing. Towards the end of the 38th week, however, the respiration becomes easier again, because the baby's head moves further down into the pelvic region. The uterus also redescends and the mother can again practise complete yogic breathing in three parts (See p. 60).

The mother usually gives birth towards the end of the 40th week, but sometimes birth takes place earlier or later than this. The fact that the baby arrives early or late does not represent a danger for mother or child, and ten to fifteen days either way will not lead to problems.

To find out the approximate date of birth, count from the first day of the last menstruation period, jump back three months and add seven days. To take an example, if the last menstruation period began on 12th January, the baby will probably arrive on 19th October of the same year, i.e. 12th January minus three months + 12th October + seven days = 19th October.

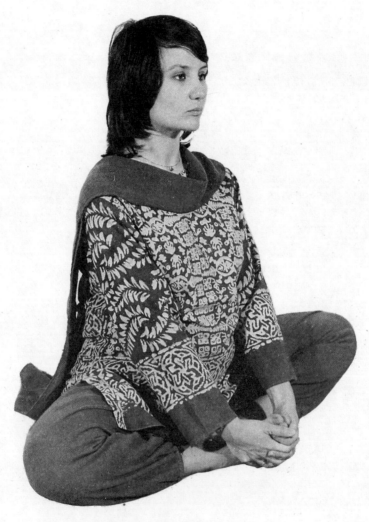

Fig. 20

For Easier Childbirth and a Healthy Baby: Asanas and Exercises During Pregnancy

The following chapters contain Anjali Devi Anand's Hathayoga course for pregnant women, based on the accumulated experience of many years' teaching at the *Centre Indien de Yoga* in Paris.

We shall now turn, therefore, to the exercises the pregnant woman should perform in order to ensure that she and her child enjoy perfect health, and that she approaches natural childbirth without fear and in the best possible easy conditions.

It is important to note, however, that not all the exercises in this chapter can be performed within the space of a single session. A choice must be made, based on the future mother's constitution and state of health, as well as the stage of development of her pregnancy. In some instances, certain postures must be performed after modifications or not performed at all.

Warning

Yoga is 100% effective and beneficial providing it is practised correctly and in strict accordance with set rules.

Pregnant women must not perform too many physical or respiratory exercises in succession, but alternate them with other asanas in order to avoid becoming tired. After each asana they should relax for a moment, either lying on their back, or on their side, or in a sitting position.

The length and number of repetitions should gradually be increased and these exercises should be practised under the guidance of an experienced instructor, skilled in the teaching of Yoga to pregnant women and who takes account of the opinions expressed by the doctor monitoring the woman's pregnancy.

The mother-to-be should not perform the exercises if she is full stomach and should wait at least four and a half hours after a full meal. Before starting the exercises, she should air the room to be used and make sure she goes to the toilet.

Relaxing on One Side and Then the Other
(Modified Savasana)

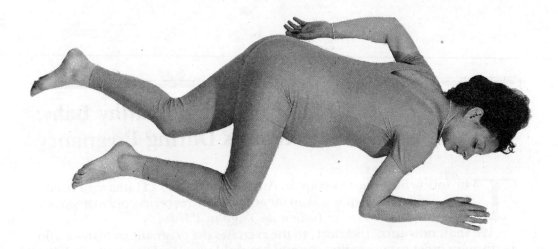

Fig. 21

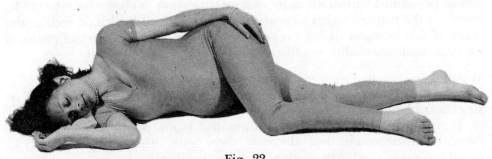

Fig. 22

Relaxing on One Side and Then the Other : (Modified Savasana)
The mother should begin by lying for a few moments first on one side and then on the other, in order to dispel fatigue. During Pregnancy, many women find they can relax more easily on their sides than on their back. This posture is usually performed during the first dilatory stages of labour.

Once she has relaxed, the mother sits up cross-legged and begins the course by gathering her thoughts for a few moments. This enables her to clear her mind of the ups and downs of everyday life, and remain alert and attentive as each exercise is performed in serenity.

Preliminary Stretching and Suppling Exercises

These exercises are designed to render suppleness to the legs and pelvic region, straighten the spinal column and stimulate the blood circulation.

They prepare the woman for meditation posture and help her to perform them more effectively, i.e. by sitting correctly—back straight, either in the *Sukhasana* cross-legged posture, *Samasana* i.e. symmetrical posture, *Ardha-Padmasana* i.e. Half-Lotus or *Padmasana* i.e. Lotus position.

The meditation postures are among the most important because in these asanas complete yogic breathing, Pranayama, interiorisation of the mind, concentration, and meditation are all performed. In these key Yogic asanas the body assumes the form of a triangle—symbolising harmony and balance.

In addition, these postures are extremely good for the entire pelvic region, and are recommended for pregnant women.

Three Exercises for Straightening
The Spinal Column

(1) *Stretching the back, legs outstretched (Uttana-asana):* Sit with the hands on the ground beside the buttocks. Curve the torso outwards by drawing back the shoulder blades. Relax. repeat the exercise two or three times in succession.

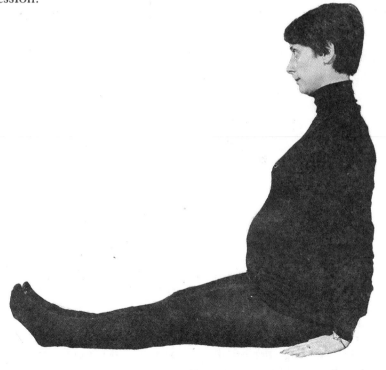

Fig. 23

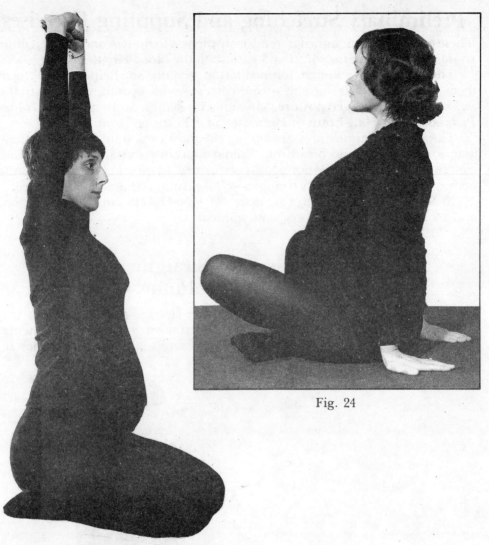

Fig. 24

Fig. 25

(2) *Stretching the back, cross-legged:* This exercise is the same as the one described in Uttana-asana, except that it is practised while sitting cross-legged.

(3) *Stretching the back, kneeling:* Begin by kneeling. Lower the body onto the feet, and interlock the hands, palms upward. Raise the arms above the head. While inhaling, straighten the back and arms. Hold this stretched position for two seconds, and retain the breath. While exhaling, relax the back and arms, keeping the hands above the head.

Perform three stretchings in succession, in co-ordination with the breathing. Round off with the posture for relaxing the back (See p. 81). We shall now turn to the exercises designed to loosen up the pelvis and legs, in preparation for the meditation postures.

50

Suppling Exercises

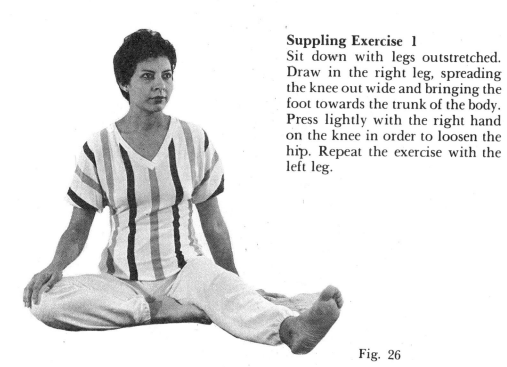

Suppling Exercise 1
Sit down with legs outstretched.
Draw in the right leg, spreading
the knee out wide and bringing the
foot towards the trunk of the body.
Press lightly with the right hand
on the knee in order to loosen the
hip. Repeat the exercise with the
left leg.

Fig. 26

Suppling Exercise 2
Adopt a sitting position and draw
in first one leg and then the other,
while at the same time spreading
the knees out wide and placing one
foot in front of the other near the
trunk of the body. Press on both
knees in order to loosen the pelvis
and legs. Repeat the exercise the
other way round.

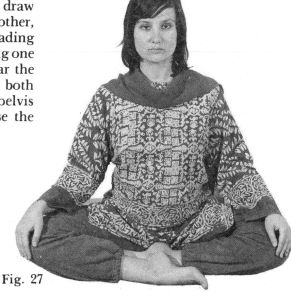

Fig. 27

Meditation Postures
1 Samasana
The Symmetrical Posture

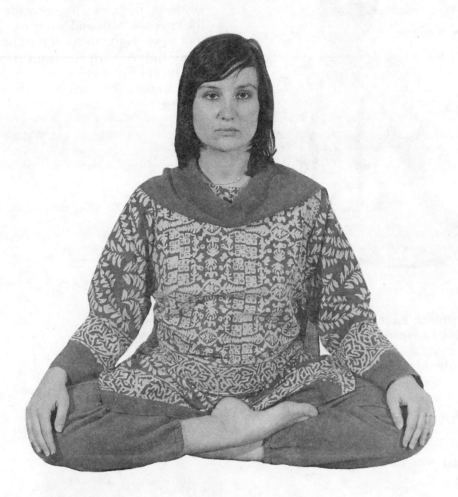

Fig. 28

1. Samasana : The Symmetrical Posture

To practise *Samasana,* begin by sitting with the legs stretched out. Bend and spread the knees, put the heel of one foot in front of the other, and, using the hands, place the first heel exactly on top of the other so that both heels are centred near the trunk of the body. The smaller toes of the upper foot are hidden between the base of the calf and the thigh of the opposite leg. The position of the heels may thereafter be reversed.

2. Ardha-Padmasana
The Half-Lotus Posture

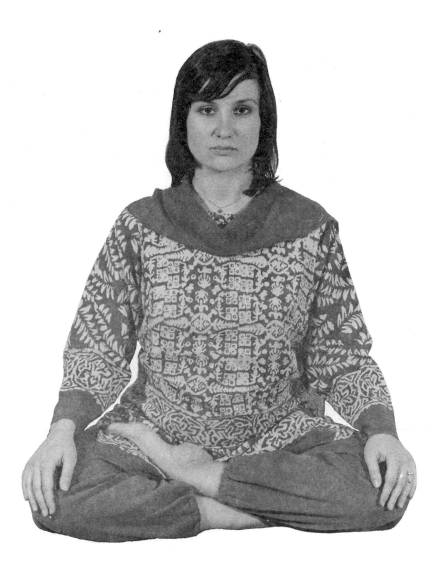

Fig. 29

2. Ardha-Padmasana : The Half-Lotus Posture
This exercise is begun in a sitting position, with the legs outstretched. Bend and spread one knee—e.g. the right one, put the foot on the ground in front of the groin of the opposite leg. Next place the heel of the left foot on the right thigh. Stay in that asana for a few moments, then reverse the position of the legs.

3. Padmasana
The Lotus Posture

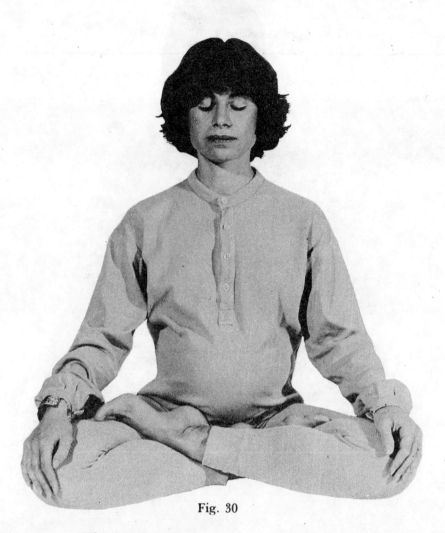

Fig. 30

3. Padmasana : The Lotus Posture

To perform this asana, begin with the legs outstretched. Bend and spread the knees, and place first the right foot on the left thigh, then the left foot on the right thigh. The full Lotus posture, also called the foot-lock, is not recommended to women who have never practised it before becoming pregnant.

4. Sukhasana
The Comfortable Posture

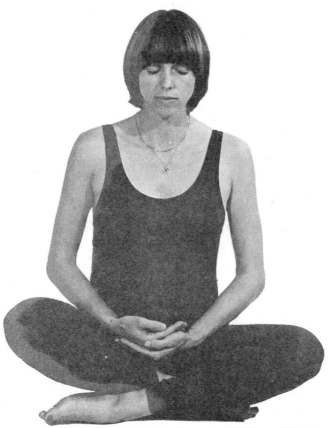

Fig. 31

4. Sukhasana : The Comfortable Posture

If the above three postures are too difficult, they can be replaced by *Sukhasana*, in which one sits cross-legged. For all meditation postures, once the legs are in position, it is important to straighten the spinal column and ensure that the back, neck and head are all in a straight line. One should then close the eyes and direct the attention within oneself, except while practising tratak (See *Kriyas* p.11)

Generally speaking, the hands should rest on the knees during the breathing exercises. During interiorisation or meditation, the back of the right hand rests in the palm of the left one.

Pregnant women should take care that they should never remain with the legs crossed for too long, so as not to block the blood circulation. Learning to perform these exercises with ease means practising them regularly, patiently, and without forcing oneself.

Exercises Specially Designed To Prepare For Childbirth

The following exercises are practised while lying on the ground

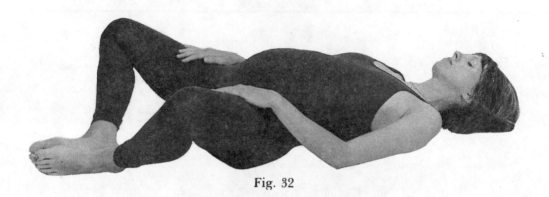

Fig. 32

(a) Bend the knees while keeping the feet together and slowly spreading out first the right leg, then the left one, then both legs together. The hands can be resting on the thighs, and slight pressure may be applied in order to supple the pelvis. In order to avoid fatigue, the lumbar region should not be arched, but should remain in contact with the ground.

(b) The same exercise can be performed with the feet crossed.

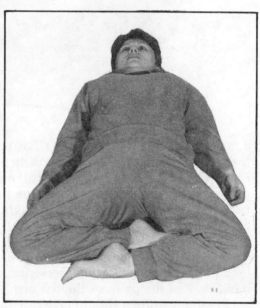

Fig. 33

56

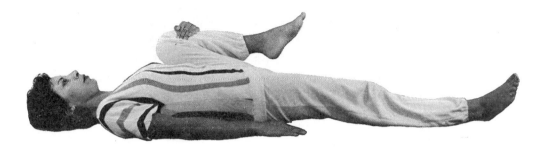

Fig. 34

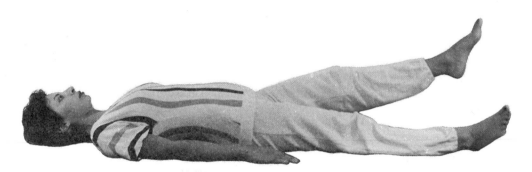

Fig. 35

(c) A different exercise performed on the back is to bend the left knee by raising and spreading it in order to bring it close to the left arm with the help of the left hand. The position is then performed on the right side. It is imperative for the pregnant woman to avoid pressing the legs against the abdomen.

(d) To practise this exercise, which contains an additional movement to strengthen the abdominal muscles, first raise one leg about 20 cm (9'') off the ground. Bend the knee and bring it close to the arm with the help of the hand. Stretch the leg out again, holding it the same distance off the floor for several seconds before lowering it to the ground. Perform the Exercise with the other leg.

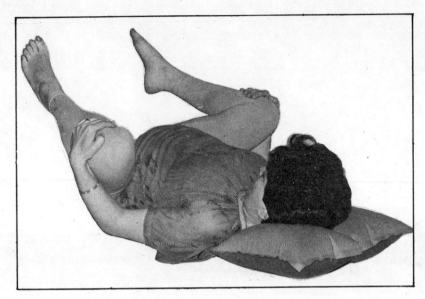

Fig. 36

(e) The same exercise can subsequently be performed using both legs, without the additional movement. This position may be used for pushing the baby down during childbirth.

(f) Merudandasana : Spinal Column Posture : Lie on the back, legs flexed, feet on the ground, and arms by the sides. Slightly raise the head and trunk. Remain in this position, with the back curved, for several seconds, then lie back and relax.

This posture trains the abdominal muscles which come into play when the baby is delivered.

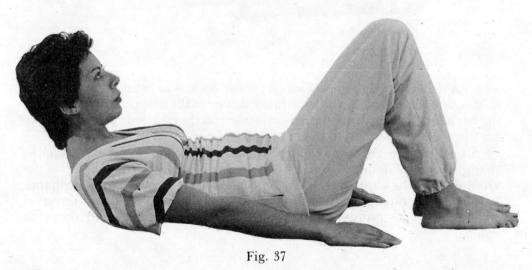

Fig. 37

(g) Another exercise is performed with the legs spread apart, knees bent, feet on the ground and with the hands grasping the ankles. Raise the head and lower the chin. This is a further position which the mother can assume during the expulsion period of labour. The forward movement of the head helps her to push the baby out.

(h) A similar exercise is practised lying on the back with the legs spread apart, knees bent and feet (especially the heels) placed on the ground. Place the arms under the legs, then grasp the top part of the inside of the thighs. Lifting the legs off the ground slightly, makes it easier to move into this posture. Indian women often adopt it to expel the child.

Each exercise may be repeated two or three times with normal breathing.

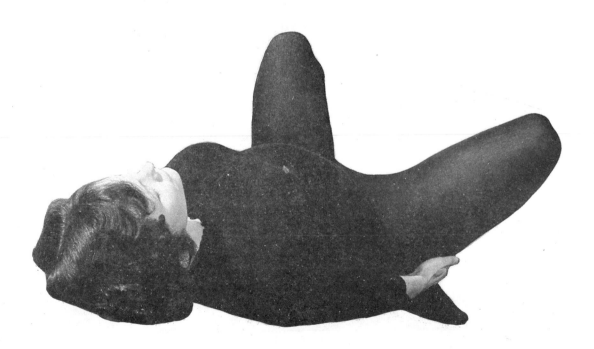

Fig. 38

Breathing Exercises

Complete Yogic Breathing

The future mother should learn how to breathe correctly and practise complete yogic breathing. This may be divided into three different levels: abdominal (diaphragm), middle-chest, and upper-chest (clavicular). The combination of these three levels of breathing constitutes complete yogic breathing. To begin with, each level of breathing is practised separately, as follows:

Abdominal Breathing

The hands may be placed (without pressing) on the umbilical region to help feel the breathing. When inhaling, gently curve the abdominal wall by lowering the diaphragm, and while exhaling, slightly contract the abdominal muscles. Breathe several times.

Middle-Chest Breathing

The hands may be lightly placed on the sides. Expand the ribs on inhaling, and contract them on exhaling—like an accordeon. Breathe several times.

Upper-Chest (Clavicular) Breathing

The collarbones may be touched with the tips of the fingers. When inhaling, slightly raise the collarbones, and lower them while exhaling. Repeat the exercise several times.

To perform complete yogic breathing, begin by exhaling, and then fill the lower part of the lungs with air by lowering the diaphragm, thereby pushing the abdominal wall forward a little. Continue inhaling by expanding the ribs, and finish by slightly raising the collar-bones. The entire inhaling process should take place with a gentle, wave-like movement.

Having filled the lungs with air, one empties them completely by slightly contracting the abdominal muscles and gradually tightening the ribs again.

This type of breathing should always take place through the nose, the air passing through the nose being warmed, humidified and purified of the dust particles it contains.

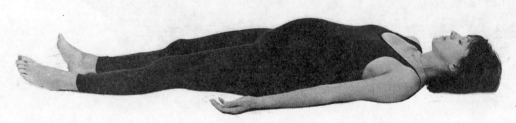

Fig. 39

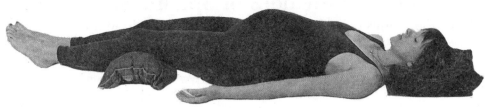

Fig. 40

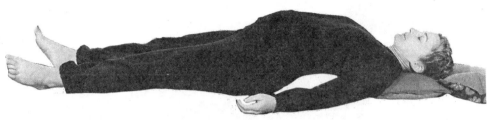

Fig. 41

Indeed, in everyday life, one should always avoid breathing through the mouth, in order to remain in good health. Breathe deeply and rhythmically, neither too quickly nor to slowly, and do not force the length of each breath. The breathing rhythm used on the present course ensures proper oxygenation and circulation, as well as the elimination of toxins. Inhalation and exhalation generally last an average of five seconds each, but if this proves uncomfortable, the rhythm should be abbreviated. Since breathing is a natural process, one should feel perfectly at ease when practising it, and should not have the impression that one is out of breath. Yogic breathing can be performed standing up (e.g. while on a walk), sitting or lying down. In the present course, it is practised in a sitting position, with the legs crossed, or while lying on the back. If performed on the back, a pillow or cushion can be put under the knees, back or head, depending on the woman's constitution and the stage of pregnancy. To avoid too great an arching of the loins, we place inflatable cushions under the thighs and the knees. (See Fig. 79)

During complete yogic breathing, concentrate the attention on the breath and feel the air rushing through the respiratory tracts. Be aware of the *prana*— the vital energy contained in the air—as it permeates every part of the body and allow it to pervade you through and through. A few deeply, rhythmically, and correctly performed respirations will charge the system with new energy and remove all feeling of fatigue, anxiety and irritability.

A pregnant woman who has learned complete yogic breathing, and knows how to control her breath, goes on practising these exercises, she will feel their beneficial effects for the rest of her life and at every level. She will have no difficulty in following the advice concerning breathing which is given to her at the moment of childbirth.

The Different Methods of Specific Respiration

These respirations ease childbirth and considerably help to alleviate labour pains. To practise these exercices, the woman should lie on her back. In order to help her feel the movement of her respiration, she can place one hand on the stomach and the other on the ribs.

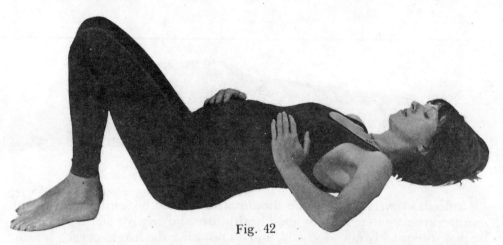

Fig. 42

The contractions of the uterus during the dilatation of the cervix require a great muscular effort and an increased supply of oxygen. Thus it is very important to know how to breathe properly and learn how to relax. If performed correctly, during contractions, relaxation helps prevent spasms of the womb.

Once the first contractions begin to take place, breathe deeply and regularly at the three different levels—complete Yogic breathing i.e.; never force or strain when inhaling or exhaling.

Once the contractions grow longer, leave aside abdominal breathing, and simply perform middle and upper-chest respiration. In the course we teach, and we make women perform middle and upper-chest breathing: slowly and deeply at first, in as much as it is possible to do so without abdominal breathing, then more quickly but still quite deeply. We round off with an exclusively upper-chest (clavicular) breathing— which is short and shallow— as always through the nose. During labour, however, at the moment of childbirth, these respirations will be more or less panting, and will often be performed through the mouth because so much air is needed that breathing through the nose is no longer sufficient.

Then follows a breathing practice which is very rapid and shallow. Although this rapid upper-chest breathing is not a yogic exercise. We mention it because it is highly valued and recommended by doctors in France not only for contractions, but as a way of diverting the attention of the woman in labour whenever she feels the need to push the child prematurely.

Once the woman has learned these breathing exercises, we move on to techniques of holding the breath, used while the mother is expelling the child.

As will be remembered, however, in Chapter 2·(p. 36), we said that those who practise Yoga uniquely for health reasons, i.e. laymen or laywomen, they should not perform retention of the breath during Pranayama. This applies even more so to pregnant women, but the specific childbirth respirations we teach in our courses are not Pranayama exercises, even though the technique is partly based on Ujjayi Pranayama. Furthermore, these specific respirations involve holding the breath for very short periods of time which, while not dangerous, are sufficient to help prepare the woman for childbirth. With full lungs, the woman in labour clearly has more strength to push the baby down, but if the breath is held too long during the preparatory exercises, this could have a disastrous effect on the baby's and the mother's health, especially if she has a weak heart or lungs, or suffers from high or low blood pressure. In cases such as these, we make women practise breathing without retention (See Exercise 3). We advise not to keep the lungs full of air for more than three to five seconds and not to repeat the exercises more than five times in any one session or day.

The following three breathing exercises are extremely useful during the phase when the mother is delivering the child, for these exercises may allow her to produce a maximum effect with a minimum expenditure of effort.

Exercise 1

"Ha.a.a..." Breathing: The woman should rest for a few moments on her side, then once again lie on her back. Next, she should bend her knees, place her legs apart and her feet on the ground at a distance of some 35 cm. To perform this exercise, her head should be resting on a thick pillow (or inflatable cushion) and should be sufficiently raised to enable the woman to press her chin on the upper part of the sternum without tiring her neck during breath retention. This forward movement of the head helps the woman to push down the baby during the expulsion period of labour

She should empty the lungs, and then perform deep, middle and upper-chest breathing through the nose. She should keep the lungs full of air for three to five seconds, with mouth shut, and completely close the glottis by contracting the neck muscles [1] and lowering the chin in order fully to retain the air. The pregnant woman should use these few seconds to practise what she will have to perform to push the baby out of the vagina. Practice involves gently contracting the abdominal muscles and at the same time making sure that the lumbar region is firmly in contact with the ground. Remember to relax the muscles of the perineum so that the baby does not encounter any resistance in its passage out of the body. **Asvinimudra (See Fig. 50)** is the best possible exercise for learning to relax the muscles of the perineum.

Exhalation takes place with the chin raised, the neck muscles relaxed, mouth open and while emitting the sound "Ha.a.a...", rather like a sigh of relief.

---

1. Do not clench the teeth.

"Ha.a.a..." breathing can be repeated two or three times, with a short period of relaxation between each respiration.

Exercise 2

Breathing partly based on the technique of Ujjayi Pranayama, with slight retention of the breath. We teach pupils Ujjayi Pranayama (See Fig. 81) in the first lessons of our course, following the yogic postures. Having learned this breathing technique, the pregnant woman should have no difficulty in performing the following exercise.

Empty the lungs. Breathe deeply through the nose—middle and upper chest—allowing the rib cage to spread fully. Hold the breath, mouth closed, for roughly four seconds. Close the glottis completely by contracting the neck muscles and lowering the chin [2] Exhale as slowly as possible through the nose, slightly loosening the neck muscles, i.e. keeping the glottis half-closed. This allows one to control the volume of air, and to use the breath to help push down the baby during labour. The partial contraction of the neck muscles produces a low continuous sound.

During daily practice, this deliberately long and continuous exhalation can usually last up to eight seconds without tiring the future mother. The purpose of the exercise is to help the mother push down on the baby for long periods, first with the lungs full,[3] then while exhaling very gradually. Throughout this exercise, the mother should try to imagine labour and, without forcing, contract the abdominal muscles which play an essential part in the pushing-down process. To make this easier, she should keep the lumbar region in contact with the ground, and avoid straining the muscles of the perineum. As noted in the previous exercise, the practice of Asvinimudra (See Fig. 50) is the best way for the pregnant woman to learn how to exert and consciously relax the muscles of the vagina. The training of the abominal and perineal muscles is a highly important step towards preparing and easing childbirth.

This breathing exercise can be repeated two or three times in succession, with a short period of relaxation between each respiration.

Exercise 3

Breathing based on the technique of Ujjayi Pranayama, but this time without retention of the breath. This exercise is performed in the same way as the previous one, except for women for whom it would be harmful to hold the breath (due to weak heart, lungs, high or low blood-pressure, etc.), hence the omission of retention.

Having emptied the lungs, inhale deeply (middle and upper chest), expanding the ribs as far as they will go. Exhale as slowly as possible through the nose. Contract the neck muscles so that the glottis is half closed, thereby ensuring that even little air is expelled at once. This will allow the pregnant woman to use her breath to push down on the child for a longer period and more easily as the baby emerges from her body. At that time if she needs to

---

2. This technique, among other beneficial effects, helps to reduce pressure on the eyeballs during the pushing.

3. During labour, as long as she can without overstrain.

inhale again, she must do so very quickly and then exhale as previously in order to continue the pushing.

As in the previous exercise, the mother should contract the abdominal muscles, without forcing, while keeping the perineal muscles relaxed during exhalation, which can last up to ten seconds. She should relax for a few seconds between each respiration. The exercise can be repeated several times in succession.

Note : While expelling the child, it is essential for the woman not to lose her breath control. It might be possible that she may not be able to retain her breath or even attempt to inhale while pushing down on the baby.

According to the doctors in India, the woman must on no account inhale while expelling the child, as this would make "breathe her baby in again." On the contrary, the above three exercises will help her to "breathe her baby out."

Through regular practice of these three exercises, the future mother learns how to control her respiration and the muscles which come into play during the bearing-down period. She will thus be well-prepared, and will have no difficulty in following the instructions of the doctor or midwife, and will stand a good chance of experiencing little, if any, pain during childbirth.

Asanas
Bhadrasana
Sitting Posture, Soles of the Feet Together

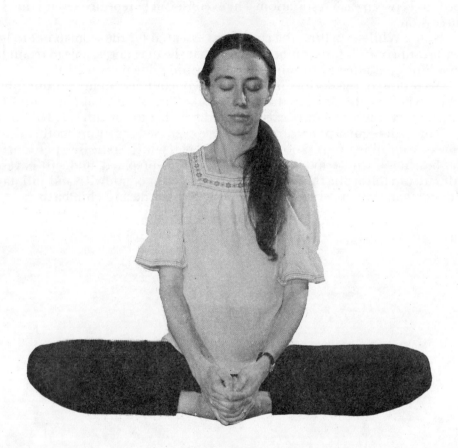

Fig. 43

Bhadrasana : Sitting Posture, Soles of the Feet Together
This posture is highly recommended by authoritative yogic texts. It is a good way of exercising the pelvis, pelvic region and hip joints, and of keeping the uro-genital system in good health. It eases childbirth and alleviates labour pains.

Adopt a sitting position, knees wide apart, and soles of the feet together. The feet should be as close to the trunk of the body as possible, and the hands crossed over the feet.

While performing this asana (which can last up to thirty seconds), keep the back straight and the knees as low as possible. Breathe regularly.

Tadasana
The Standing Posture

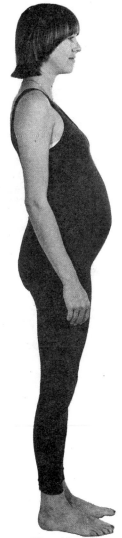

Fig. 44

Tadasana : The Standing Posture

This posture is performed in standing position, with the spinal column very straight, keeping arms on one's sides, and feet slightly apart. The buttock muscles should be tensed and relaxed several times in succession during this exercise. While the buttock muscles are being contracted, the pelvis is tilted forward slightly. This prevents the future mother from arching the loins and ensures that she does not become fatigued or subject to pain while standing.

Utkatasana
The Squatting Posture

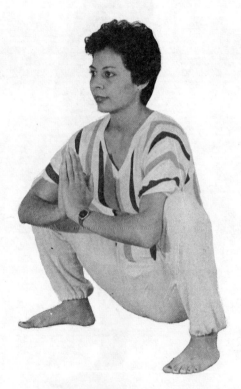

Fig. 45

Utkatasana: The Squatting Posture

This exercise is performed with the legs apart, feet parallel, and heels on the ground. Begin by slowly bending the knees and squatting with the lower part of the buttocks in line with the ankles. Join the palms of the hands and position the elbows between the knees to help keep them apart. Hold this posture for a few moments, then stand up again. Should this *asana* prove difficult for those who have no practice in it, they should support themselves against a piece of furniture or ask someone to help them.

This exercise can be repeated two or three times. Breathe regularly and direct your attention towards the pelvic region. The squatting posture helps prepare the woman for childbirth, for it is similar to the position she will assume on her back during labour and delivery. Indeed, in many countries, certain women adopt a squatting position to give birth to their child. This asana exercises and tones up the pelvis and legs, and alleviates pain in the lumbar region. In the later stages of pregnancy, however, this asana should be avoided as soon as the mother experiences the slightest feeling of fatigue.

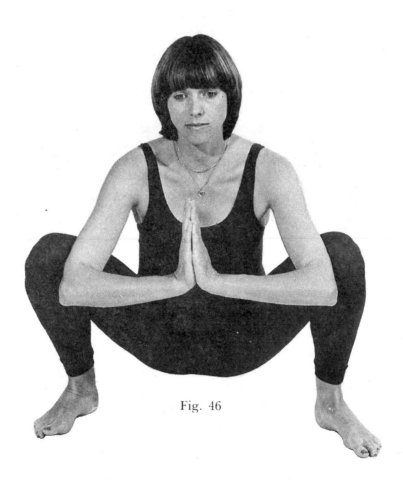

Fig. 46

Utkatasana

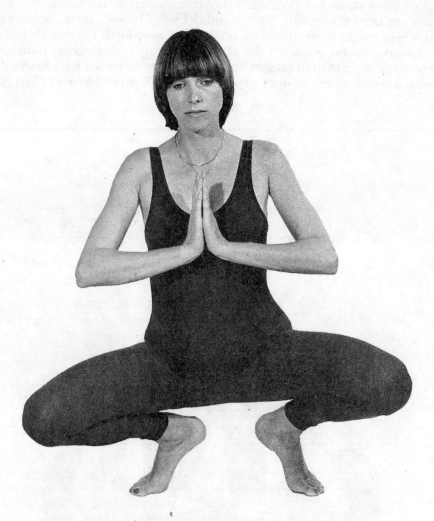

Fig. 47

Utkatasana : A Variation

This variation is performed by bending and spreading the knees wide apart, crouching on the tips of the toes, heels not too far apart, and placing the joined hands in front of the chest. Should one experience the slightest difficulty, it is advisable either to prop oneself up against a piece of furniture or get help from someone else.

This asana should be repeated two or three times for several seconds. Breathe regularly and direct the concentration towards the pelvis. The posture strengthens the legs, improves blood circulation and is beneficial to the pelvic region. The same exceptions apply as for the previous asana.

Paschimottanasana (Modified)
Modified Posterior Stretching Posture

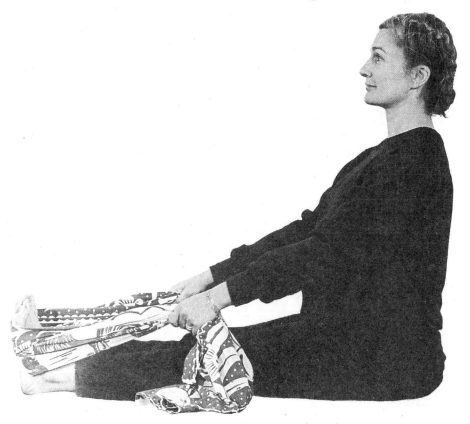

Fig. 48

Paschimottanasana (Modified) : Modified Posterior Stretching Posture
It is not possible to bend the trunk close to the thighs, or lie on the stomach
during pregnancy. Certain yogic postures must therefore be modified, but this
in no way detracts from their unquestionable beneficial effects. (See Fig. 11)

The future mother adopts a sitting position, and uses a scarf or towel to
stretch the back and legs. To be quite, certain that the legs are fully
outstretched, raise the heels two cms above the ground. Lower the shoulders,
bring the shoulder blades closer together, and straighten up the spinal
column. Hold the position for a few seconds, then relax. Repeat the exercise
two or three times in succession. Breathe regularly. Concentrate on the back
and legs.

This modified asana tones the body, and is good for the sacro-lumbar
region, spinal column and sciatic nerve. It soothes the pain often felt in the
back during pregnancy and helps remedy inward curvature of the spine called
lordosis.

71

Janusirasana (Modified)
Modified Head-Touching-Knee Posture

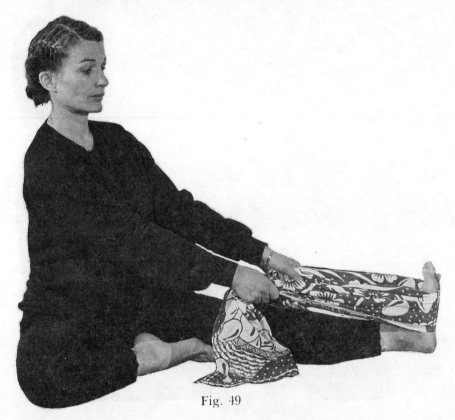

Fig. 49

Janusirasana (Modified) : Modified Head-Touching-Knee Posture
Practise this exercise in a sitting position, one leg completely outstretched, the other with the knee bent outwards and the heel close to the perineum. As in the Paschimottanasana, use a towel to help stretching, and be sure to keep the back very straight. Until the fifth month, this exercise and the previous one can be practised without the help of a scarf or towel. Grip the feet with the hands, i.e. with the thumb and index finger round the big toe, like a pincer, (See photographs of Paschimottanasana and Janusirasana). During pregnancy, however, instead of bending the torso towards the legs, straighten the back by means of an upward movement.

This asana should be practised on either side for several seconds, two or three times in succession. One should breathe regularly and direct the concentration to the sacro-lumbar region. The exercise produces beneficial effects similar to those of Paschimottanasana, but the stretching of the sacro-lumbar region is more powerful on the side where the knee is bent. Janusirasana tones up the hips and improves the circulation in the pelvic region.

72

Asvini-Mudra in Januvaksasana
Symbol of the Mare in the Knee-Chest Posture

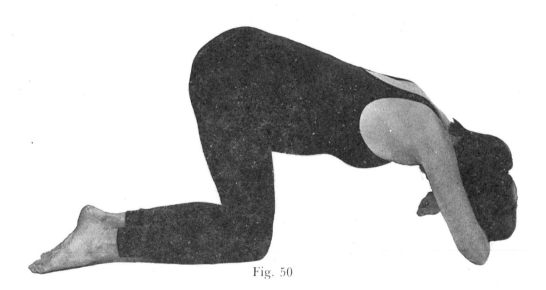

Fig. 50

Asvini-Mudra in Januvaksasana : Symbol of the Mare in the Knee-Chest Posture

This asana involves the contraction and relaxation of the buttock muscles, sphyncter, perineum, and the entire pelvic region. It is one of the most important exercises for preparing the mother for childbirth. It is performed with the knees slightly apart, and the forehead resting on the arms folded on the ground.

While inhaling, consciously relax the muscles of the entire pelvic region and gradually contract them while exhaling. Keep the lungs empty for one second, with the muscles of the pelvic region contracted as tightly as possible, then inhale again while at the same time fully relaxing the muscles. Breathe rhythmically—four or five seconds each for inhalation and exhalation.

In the course we teach for pregnant women, we slightly modify the breathing used in this Mudra so that it is more suited to the specific breathing exercises designed for childbirth (See Exercises on pp. 63-64). These exercises are performed by relaxing the muscles of the perineum during exhalation; we have therefore decided to adopt the same principle.

Modified Asvinimudra is performed as follows: Inhale and exhale while consciously relaxing the muscles of the entire pelvic region and perineum. Keep the lungs empty for three or four seconds while gradually contracting the muscles of the pelvic region. Completely relax these same muscles while performing a further inhalation and exhalation. Pay special attention to the muscles of the vagina (perineum), and ensure that the breathing, while fairly rapid—roughly three or four seconds each for inhaling and exhaling—is deep and rhythmic.

One should repeat Asvinimudra (whether modified or not) three to five times in succession. Next, one should relax, and if one shows no signs of fatigue, start all over again. The concentration should be directed towards the pelvic region, but first and foremost, to the perineum.

Regular practice of this Mudra exercises and strengthens the muscles of entire pelvic region. It helps the mother cope with the weight of the child during pregnancy and eases childbirth by virtue of the fact that the mother is perfectly trained in relaxing the muscles of the vagina. The woman in labour creates no resistance, and therefore saves herself pain and fatigue.

This posture is recommended in cases of retroversion or descent of the uterus. This is also an excellent posture for soothing pains in the lumbar region and for supplying fresh blood to the brain.

Those with high or low blood pressure should take care while practising Asvinimudra in the Januvaksasana i.e. knee-chest posture. The Asvinimudra for contraction and relaxation of the pelvic muscles can also be practised while lying on the back with the knees bent.

Chakrasana
Modified Wheel Posture on the Ground

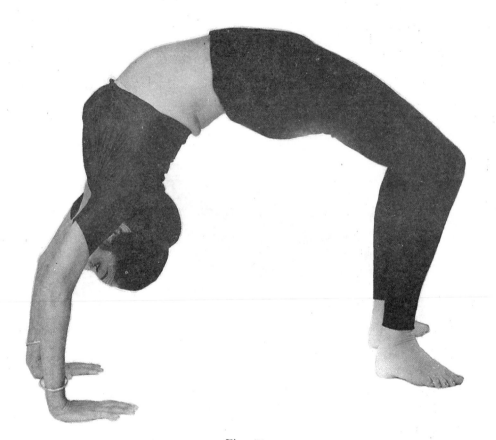

Fig. 51

Chakrasana : Modified Wheel Posture on the Ground

This posture has been considerably simplified. Lie on the back with arms by the sides, the palms of the hands against the ground, knees bent, and feet drawn in near the trunk of the body.

Raise the pelvis, contract the buttock muscles for a few seconds, then rest the back on the ground. Breathe regularly and direct the concentration to the pelvic region. Repeat the exercise two or three times in succession.

This posture exercises the lower part of the spinal column, and tones the muscles of the pelvic region and thighs. It helps alleviate pains in the abdomen caused by the weight of the foetus.

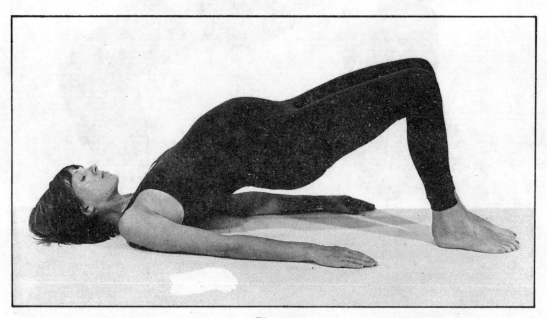

Fig. 52

Ardha-Halasana
The Half-Plough Posture

Ardha-Halasana
The Half-Plough Posture

Lie on the back with the arms and palms of the hands on the ground. Very slowly raise the legs, 30 cms at a time, holding each successive stage for a few seconds until the legs are perpendicular to the trunk of the body. Remain in this posture for five seconds, then slowly lower the legs, 30 cms at a time. Avoid arching the lumbar region, and do not use the back for support during the exercise. This asana should only be performed during the early stages of pregnancy, and is to be avoided by those suffering from lordosis i.e. inward curvature of the spine causing spondylitis etc. In order to prevent tiredness, we advise raising the legs one after the other, rather than together.

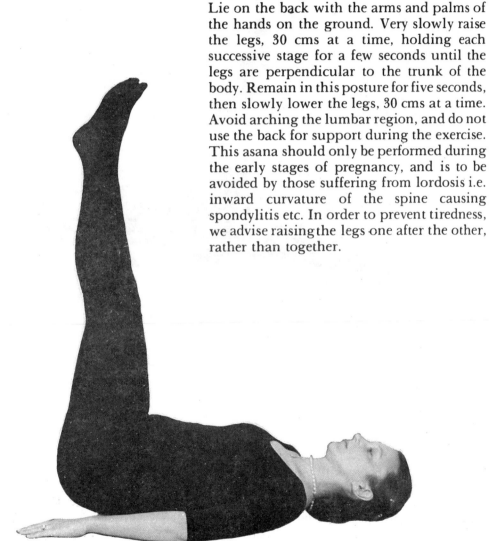

Fig. 53

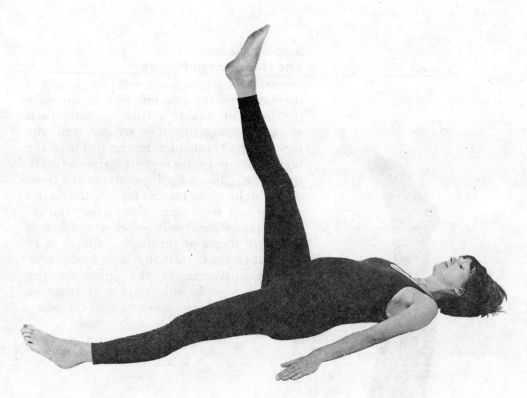

Fig. 54

This exercise can be practised twice on either side. It serves mainly to strengthen the abdominal muscles and prevent constipation by stimulating the functioning of the intestines. Breathe regularly and direct the concentration towards the abdominal region.

Ustrasana
The Camel Posture

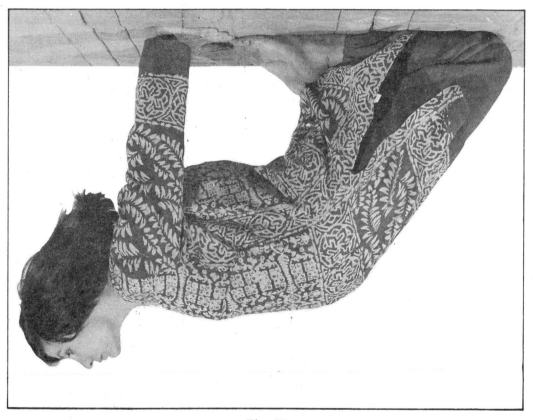

Fig. 55

Ustrasana : The Camel Posture
Take a kneeling position and sit on the feet. Drop the arms down behind the body, hands on the ground and fingers prolonging the line of the feet. While inhaling, raise the trunk, arch the torso upwards and throw the head backwards. Hold the position for two or three seconds, then while exhaling, come back to the original position and finish off in the Posture for Relaxing the Back (See next posture).

Repeat the exercise two or three times, and direct the attention towards the trunk and spinal column.

In the later stages of pregnancy, or in cases where even the slightest difficulty is encountered in performing the exercise, modify the asana by arching only the back while continuing to sit on the feet.

This posture exercises the abdominal muscles by stretching them, and stimulates the functioning of the intestines. It is recommended in cases of cyphosis (a hunch-like deformation) and stooping, and helps develop the chest. This *asana* improves blood circulation in the legs and thighs.

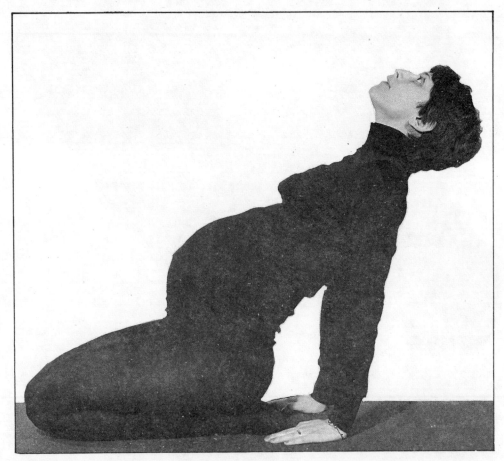

Fig. 56

Posture For Relaxing The Back

Begin by sitting on the feet with the knees apart. Slowly lean the trunk forwards until the forehead is resting on the ground.

This forward counter-movement of the previous posture helps relax the back, lumbar region, neck and head. The influx of fresh blood clears away fatigue from the brain and face.

As of the sixth month, and even before, should too much blood flow to the head, rest it on the hands rather than on the ground.

Relax completely during this posture and maintain it for five to thirty seconds maximum. Breathe regularly and direct the concentration towards relaxing the back and head.

This posture is not recommended to those suffering from high blood pressure, heartburn or feeling of nausea nor should this form of relaxation be performed while digesting food.

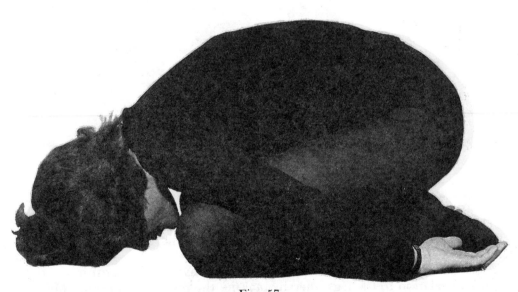

Fig. 57

Vakrasana Modified
The Modified Spinal Twist

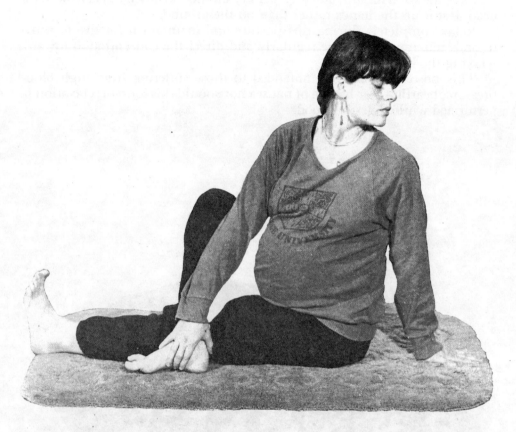

Fig. 58

Vakrasana Modified : The Modified Spinal Twist
Vakrasana was introduced into Hathayoga by Swami Kuvalyananda. It is a simplified posture performed in preparation for the exercise which is to follow, i.e. Ardha-Matsyendrasana.

We have modified both of these postures by inverting the position of the trunk in relation to the legs, thereby making the postures more suitable for mothers-to-be. The latter will be able to perform these spinal-twist asanas without being hampered by pressure on the abdominal region. Even though the positions are slightly less effective as a result of the modification, they are still very good for the spinal column and the kidneys.

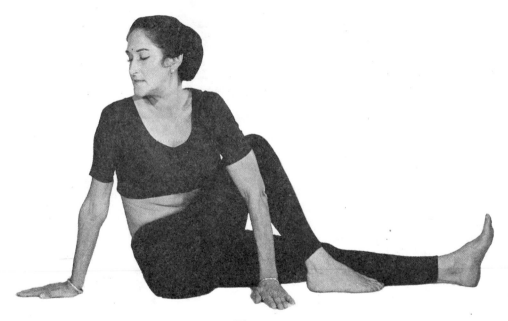

Fig. 59

Sit with the left leg outstretched, the right leg folded over it, and place the right foot flat on the ground near the knee. Hold the right foot in the right hand. Twist to the left, keeping the other hand on the ground. Make sure that the outstretched leg and the left hand are in line with one another. The shoulders and chin should follow the same line, with the chin placed above the left shoulder. Reverse the posture, practise twice on each side, for five to fifteen seconds. Breathe regularly, and direct the concentration towards the spinal column and kidneys.

Ardha-Matsyendrasana (Modified)
The Half-Matsyendra Posture

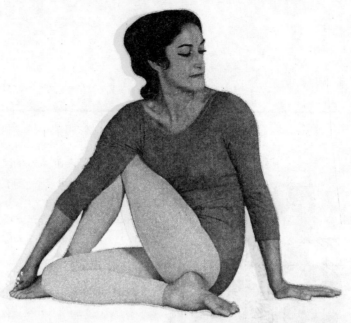

Fig. 60

In this posture, the leg is folded inwards instead of outstretched. During twists performed in the final stages of pregnancy, the weight of the body rests mainly on one buttock, bcause the centre of gravity is displaced.

The posture should be performed twice on either side for five to fifteen seconds. The breathing should remain regular, and the concentration directed towards the spinal column and the kidneys.

The pregnant woman should choose from these two postures the one most suited to her needs. To increase their beneficial effect on the spinal column, these twists should be combined with other asanas e.g. Ustrasana and Catuspadasana.

Fig. 61

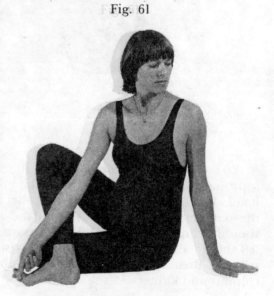

84

Catuspadasana
The Cat or All-Fours Posture

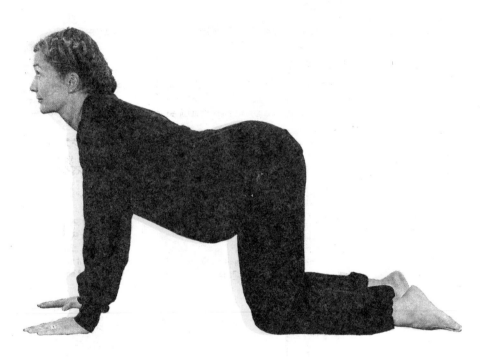

Fig. 62

Catuspadasana: The Cat or All-Fours Posture

Assume an all-fours position, with palms, knees and feet slightly apart, arms and thighs perpendicular to the ground. Inhale, hollow the small of the back, and bring the shoulder blades close together, while raising the head. Exhale, lowering the head and hunching the back.

Perform the exercise slowly, four or five times in succession, breathing regularly and directing the concentration towards the spinal column.

This posture makes the back more supple and frees it form fatigue, while at the same time soothing back pains. It helps correct uterine retroversion, which accounts for the fact that this posture is recommended not only before but after childbirth.

During pregnancy, it can partly replace the postures—such as the Cobra (*Bhujangasana*)—which a future mother cannot perform because they involve lying on the stomach.

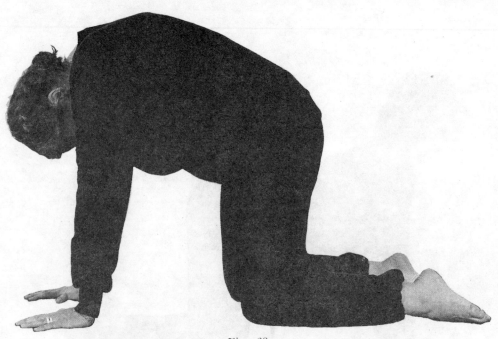

Fig. 63

Asanas for Mothers-to-be Having Practised Yogic Physical Exercises Before Pregnancy

At this point, we should like to include seven asanas reserved for pregnant women who have for long practised Yogic postures and who wish to keep fit during pregnancy. We have mainly chosen exercises for the legs and spinal column. They can be practised by future mothers who feel full of energy, but only on condition that they do not lead to fatigue. The exercises should be alternated with relaxation, and performed under the guidance of a Yoga expert. They should not be practised during the final stages of pregnancy.

1. Uttha Chakrasana

Standing Wheel Posture

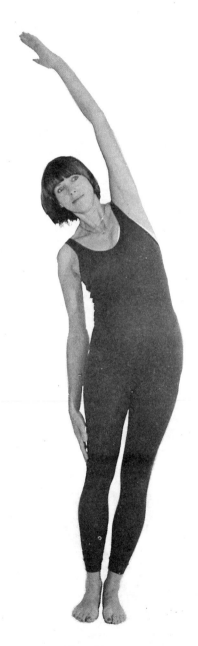

1. Uttha Chakrasana :
The Standing Wheel Posture
Stand straight, with the feet together on the ground. Raise the left arm and slowly lean to the right, sliding the right arm down the right leg. Stand up straight again, and change the position of the arms by performing a wheel-like rotation. Repeat the exercise in the reverse position. Make sure to maintain regular breathing. This asana is very good for rendering the spinal column more supple.

It also helps remedy scapular asymmetry—in this case, the posture should be performed by stretching on the side where the shoulder is too low—and prevents the formation of cellulitis—inflammation of the cellular tissue—around the waist. The posture can be repeated two or three times, with regular breathing and the concentration directed towards the spinal column.

Fig. 64

2. Trikonasana
The Triangle Posture

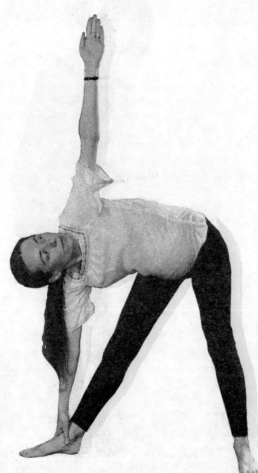

Fig. 65

2. Trikonasana : The Triangle Posture

Assume a standing position, legs apart. Inhale deeply while raising the arms to a horizontal position, then exhale while bending the trunk downwards to the right, at the same time fixing the eyes on the arm as it moves downwards until the fingers of the right hand are touching the right ankle. Make sure the right foot is slightly turned outwards. Once the arms form a vertical line, turn the head and look upwards.

Hold the position for a few moments, then inhale while resuming the standing position. Repeat the same movement, this time on the left side. Round off the exercise by exhaling and lowering the arms.

The posture should be repeated two or three times on either side, with the concentration directed to the movements of the body.

Trikonasana helps fight constipation, exercises the spinal column, especially at the hips and renders the legs more supple.

3. Padahastasana (Modified)
Back Stretching Posture, Hands on the Ground, Feet Apart

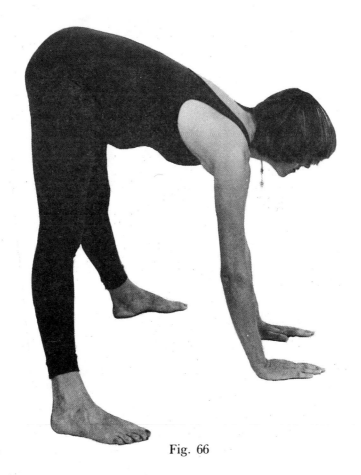

Fig. 66

3. Padahastasana (Modified) : Back Stretching Posture,
Hands on the Ground, Feet Apart
Stand with the legs wide apart. While breathing in, raise the arms, and while breathing out, slowly lean the trunk forward and place the palms of the hands on the ground. Raise the head and arch the back for several seconds while breathing in and out, then lower the head and relax. Next, raise the head and trunk while keeping the back as straight as possible and inhaling deeply. Having assumed an upright position, stretch the arms above the head, and while exhaling, lower the arms and relax standing up, feet together.

Repeat this asana two or three times, directing the concentration towards the spinal column. Modified Padahastasana is an excellent way of relieving lumbar fatigue, strengthening the back, and making the legs more supple.

89

4. Parighasana
The Cross-bar Posture (Modified)

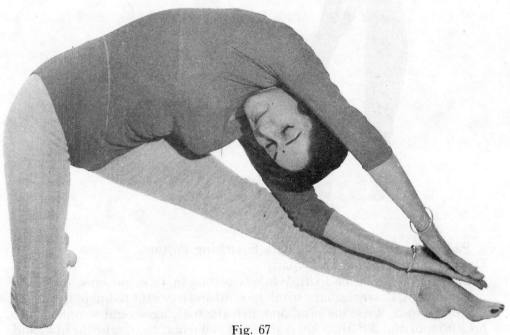

Fig. 67

4 . Parighasana : The Cross-bar Posture (Modified)

Take up a kneeling position, then stretch out the right leg, making sure to balance the weight of the body on the left leg. Inhale, while raising the arms to a horizontal position. Turn the palms of the hands upwards, and exhale while leaning the trunk towards the side with the outstretched leg. Place the back of the hand on the ankle and slowly bring the left arm over the left ear. During pregnancy, do not attempt to join the two hands. Hold the position for several seconds while breathing regularly. While inhaling, bring the trunk back to the vertical position, and while exhaling, lower the arms. Repeat the exercise on the other side.

This asana can be practised two or three times on either side, with the concentration directed towards the spinal column and the movement of the body. Parighasana is excellent for rendering the back, hips and legs more supple.

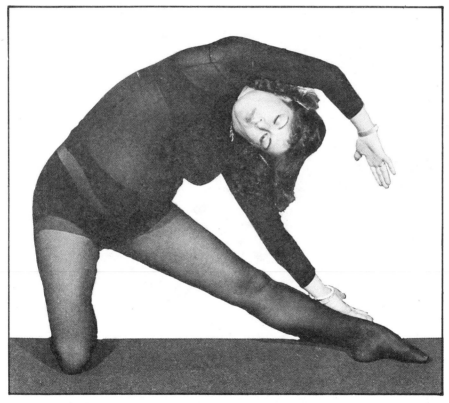

Fig. 68

5. Ardha-Bhujangasana
The Half-Cobra Posture

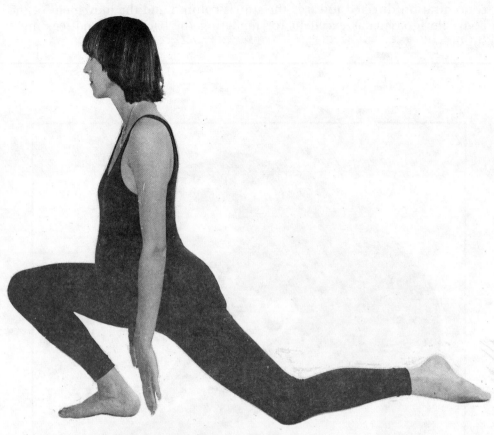

Fig. 69

5. Ardha-Bhujangasana : The Half-Cobra Posture

In a kneeling position, advance the right foot until the lower leg—having tibia and fibula bones—is perpendicular to the ground. Keep the back straight, arms by the sides, and inhale. Next, exhale while moving the weight of the body forwards and maintaining an upright position of the trunk. Bend the knee as much as possible while keeping the heel firmly on the ground. Inhale, while at the same time returning to the initial posture.

This asana should be practised twice on either side, while the concentration is directed towards the spinal column and the movement of the body. *Ardha-Bhujangasana* is an effective way of making the spinal column, legs, knees and ankles more supple.

6. Gomukhasana
The Cow Head Posture

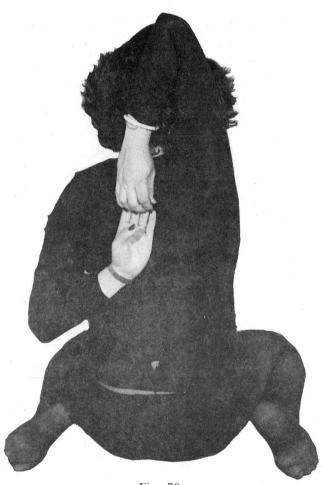

Fig. 70

6. Gomukhasana : The Cow Head Posture
Sit between the feet. Raise the right hand over the right shoulder and grasp the left hand behind the back. Be careful not to tense the neck.

Repeat the posture once or twice on either side for thirty seconds, breathing regularly and directing the concentration towards the trunk and arms. This asana has a beneficial effect on the arm and back muscles, in which it improves the blood circulation. It increases the capacity of the chest and vigorously exercises the knee joints.

93

7. Vrksasana
The Tree Posture

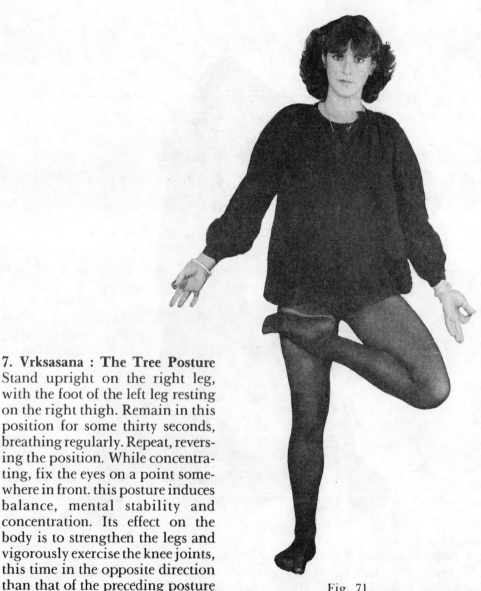

7. Vrksasana : The Tree Posture
Stand upright on the right leg, with the foot of the left leg resting on the right thigh. Remain in this position for some thirty seconds, breathing regularly. Repeat, reversing the position. While concentrating, fix the eyes on a point somewhere in front. this posture induces balance, mental stability and concentration. Its effect on the body is to strengthen the legs and vigorously exercise the knee joints, this time in the opposite direction than that of the preceding posture i.e. Gomukhasana.

Fig. 71

By selecting from these seven additional postures and combining them with the exercises already practised on a regular basis by future mothers following our course, women who are active and fit will posses complete mastery over their body. We shall now return to our normal asanas.

Relaxation, Feet Raised

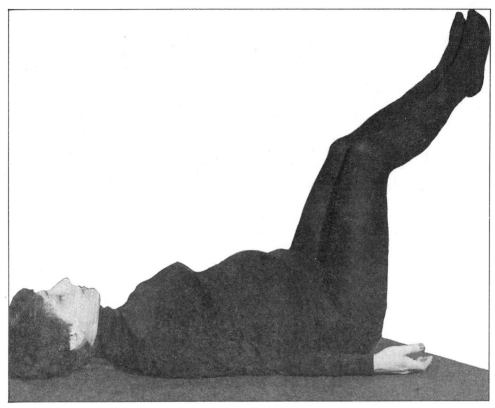

Fig. 72

Relaxation, Feet Raised

Begin by lying on the ground, legs raised, knees bent, feet against the wall, buttocks 30-40 cms away from it. Do not bring the thighs too near the abdomen, for this will block blood circulation in the groin region. Make sure the back, neck and head are in a straight line, with the chin slightly lowered in order to avoid arching the neck and tightening the cervical vertebrae. Keep the arms at a slight distance from the trunk, if possible with the palms of the hands turned upward, thus resting the shoulder blades properly on the ground. Before relaxing spend a few seconds straightening the shoulders as if to fix them to the ground. This is very beneficial to people with a bad posture, i.e. hollowed chest and stooping shoulders. To remedy an overly arched small of the back, press at the same time the lumbar region against the ground, a movement which is helped by the raised position of the feet. Having thus stretched the neck and the back, close the eyes and relax completely.

This relaxation exercise refreshes the back, small of the back, and legs. It helps decongest swollen ankles and feet, and relieves varicose veins.

Important Note

We now turn to the inverted postures, i.e. Viparita Karani and Sarvangasana. These are very important to the health because they produce a revitalising effect on the entire body. Although recommended, these postures are difficult to perform during pregnancy and can only be executed by women who have practised them over a long period. Even for those who are well-experienced in these asanas the problem is how to raise the legs and trunk without bouncing backwards the whole lower part of the body and hitting the abdomen with the thighs or pressing down on the abdominal region—all of which is dangerous for pregnant women. To help all future mothers—even those who have never before practised Hathayoga–perform these inverted positions without danger, we have modified the exercises. It is vital, however, to respect the restrictions of these asanas, detailed below. The modification consists in keeping the feet against the wall throughout the entire exercise, which enables one to perform the asana without straining and without risk of loosing one's balance. These exercises should be performed as follows:

Viparita Karani (Modified)
Modified Inverted Position

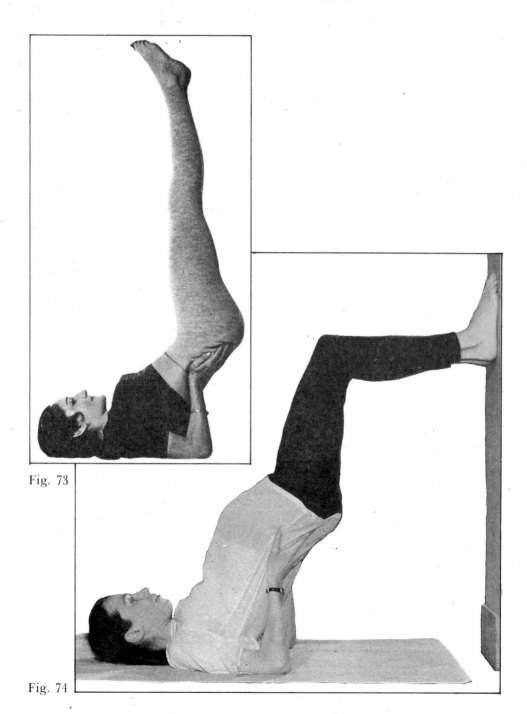

Fig. 73

Fig. 74

Viparita Karani (Modified) : Modified Inverted Position

Mothers-to-be who have just performed the Relaxation exercise and Feet Raised , will already be in the starting position. They should simply come slightly closer to the wall and bring the arms to the sides, palms to the ground. Inhale deeply at the three levels, then while exhaling, slowly raise the pelvis as high as possible by pushing with the feet against the wall. Support the hips with the hands and hold the position for as long as it is comfortable. Only abdominal breathing should be performed. Slowly lower the pelvis to the ground again, and while lying on the back, relax. Perform the exercise once or twice in succession for five to thirty seconds, slowly increasing the duration of time by five seconds a week and practising daily. Direct the concentration towards the head and neck region.

Despite the modification, Viparita Karani helps correct the hypo-or hyper-functioning of the thyroid gland, and produces a highly beneficial effect on the pituitary gland. It irrigates the brain, revitalises the nervous system, and keeps the digestive organs healthy by draining out venous blood and ensuring a richer supply of arterial blood. It helps relieve fatigue, insomnia and overtiredness, decongests the legs and feet, and helps fight varicose veins. It also makes it possible to relax the lower abdominal muscles which bear the weight of the foetus and soothes the pain which the weight can cause. This posture is of help in remedying the downward displacement of the womb.

The exercise should not be performed by women suffering from high blood-pressure, heartburn or by those who are carrying the child very high, i.e. usually from the end of the 36th week until the end of the 38th week, if it is the first child.

Sarvangasana
Modified Shoulder Stand

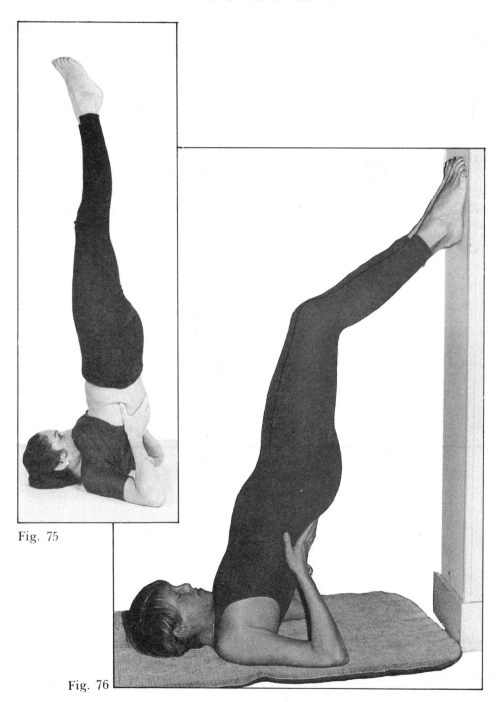

Fig. 75

Fig. 76

Sarvangasana : Modified Shoulder Stand

It is best to learn the previous exercise, first Viparita Karani, before moving on to the practice of Sarvangasana. The difference between the two asanas is that during Sarvangasana, the position of the body is more vertical. Before raising the legs and trunk, bring the lower part of the body as near as possible to the wall, even touching it. To do this, lie on the side, then turn the trunk so that it is facing the wall. With the feet against the wall, the legs should be slightly bent and spread apart to avoid pressing on the abdomen.

Inhale deeply at the three levels, then while exhaling, slowly raise the pelvis and trunk until the latter are vertical. Keep the legs slightly bent and the feet against the wall. The chin should press into the jugular knot—i.e. of the throat—just above the breastbone; this is another difference between Sarvangasana and Viparita Karani.

During Sarvangasana, breathe only at the abdominal level. Next, slowly bring the pelvis to the ground again and lie on the back to relax. This exercise may be repeated twice for five to thirty seconds, gradually increasing the time spent on it. Direct the attention to the thyroid gland.

Sarvangasana and Viparita Karani produce similar therapeutic effects on the body and the endocrine glands, but Sarvangasana has a more pronounced effect on the thyroid. Like the previous exercise, Sarvangasana is of benefit when there is downward displacement of the womb. It relaxes the abdominal muscles which support the weight of the foetus and relieves the pain caused by it. Sarvangasana and Viparita Karani produce similar therapeutic effects on the body and the endocrine glands, but Sarvangasana has a more pronounced effect on the thyroid. Like the previous exercise, Sarvangasana is of benefit when there is downward displacement of the womb. It relaxes the abdominal muscles which support the weight of the foetus and relieves the pain caused by it.

Both of these postures are wellknown for their rejuvenating power. They improve the circulation in the head and face, prevent or palliate the formation of wrinkles, combat fatigue, and are recommended to those who do not sleep well.

They are not recommended to women with high blood-pressure, heartburn or to those carrying the child very high, i.e. usually between the end of the 36th week and the end of the 38th, especially if it is the woman's first child.

Matsyasana
The Fish Posture

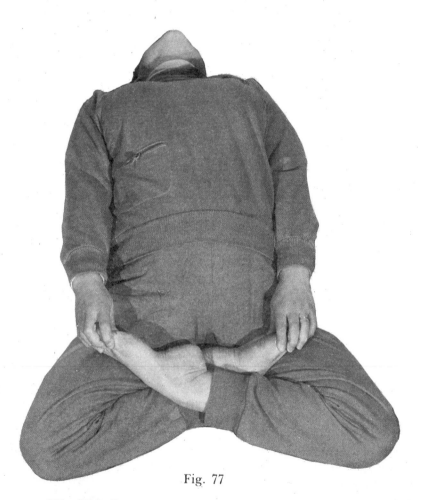

Fig. 77

Matsyasana : The Fish Posture
Sit with the legs in the Lotus position (foot-locked) and then lie on the back.
Next, lean on the elbows, raise the trunk and the head and rest the crown of the
head on the ground. Keep the spine arched and hold the big toes with the
fingers. Breathe regularly, and direct the concentration towards the thyroid
gland and neck. Each time Matsyasana should be performed for five to twenty
seconds.

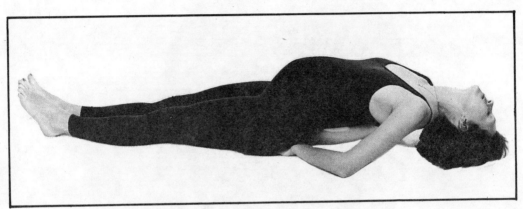

Fig. 78

This posture is complementary to Sarvangasana because it tones up the thyroid gland by exercising the neck in the reverse direction from the previous posture. If Sarvangasana and Matsyasana are practised one after the other, Matsyasana should last 1/3 of the time spent on Sarvangasana.

This Fish Posture stimulates blood circulation in the throat neck and back, and corrects cyphosis. It also fights constipation and is good for the sciatic nerve.

A more easily practised variation of this asana is to lie on the ground, legs straight, hands (with palms on the ground) under the buttocks. Supporting the trunk on the elbows, raise it and throw the head backwards and rest the crown of the head on the ground. The spine and the neck must be well arched. The Fish Posture should not be practised by those suffering from a hyperactive thyroid gland or constriction of the cervical vertebrae.

Savasana
The Complete Relaxation Posture

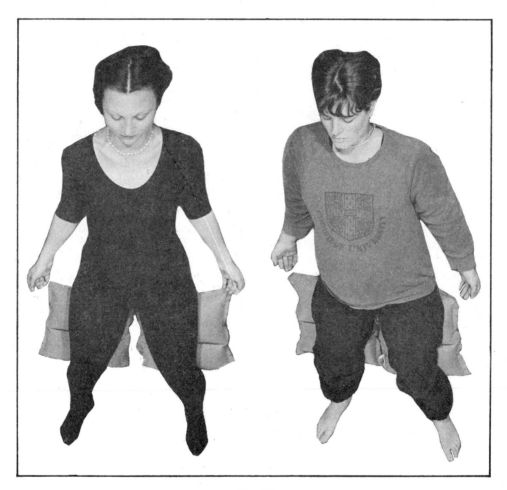

Fig. 79

Savasana : The Complete Relaxation Posture
Lie supine with the back, neck and head in a straight line. Make sure the legs and arms are slightly spread apart, with the palms of the hands partially turned upwards. According to the future mother's constitution, and during the later stages of pregnancy, it is advisable to place a small cushion under the head and a larger one under each leg, making sure, however, that the feet rest on the ground.

As already mentioned, on our course we use inflatable cushions placed under the knees and thighs so that both are sufficiently raised to avoid arching the small of the back and to help stretch the spinal column on the ground.

Phase 1: Close the eyes and relax completely. Relax the region of the thorax and listen to the regular beating of the heart. Relax the abdominal region, legs, thighs, knees, calves, ankles and feet. Next, relax the arms, shoulders, elbows, hands and fingers. Finally, relax the neck, back of the neck, head, face, forehead, eyes, eyelids, nostrils, jaws and cheeks.

Phase 2: Simultaneously relax the thoracic and abdominal regions, the legs and arms, the back of the neck i.e. the cervical region and the head.

Phase 3: Relax from head to toe, releasing each muscle, cell and nervous fibre, and allowing the weight of the body to lie on the ground. Let the feeling of weight off the entire body by withdrawing the consciousness from it.

Phase 4: Relax the mind by directing the attention uniquely to the breath. Breathe slowly, deeply and regularly, i.e. complete Yogic breathing, without ever trying to force the rhythm. Allow the breath to come and go harmoniously, while feeling the ebb and flow of each respiration. With each breath, sense that your entire being is filled with calm and well-being.

People often harbour mistaken ideas concerning Yogic relaxation, for they associate it with a kind of mental drowsiness. In fact, however, the mind should not be allowed either to wander or to fall asleep. It is important to remain consciously aware of deep relaxation. The relaxation of the body begins in the mind. If the attention wanders, it must be gently brought back, without forcing, towards the regularity of breathing, in order to avoid any thought which might trouble the mind and thereby tense the body. It is important also to make sure that one does not fall asleep, if one wants to learn to relax the mind properly for even during sleep, the mind can be troubled.

During conscious relaxation, however, when the mind identifies with no other thought but calmness, relaxation and well-being, the body and mind are truly rested.

To perform this exercise correctly, begin by practising it for short periods. Five minutes—including the four phases of relaxation—are enough. It should be practised every day and the length of time spent on it gradually increased. It should not be prolonged beyond ten minutes, but can be performed two or three times a day. After several minutes of deep relaxation, one should turn on the side and continue to relax for a few moments.

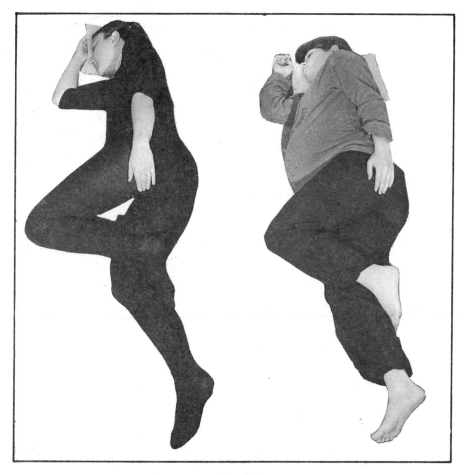

Fig. 80

Once the relaxation is over, slowly open the eyes and sit up from the right side. Complete Yogic relaxation with regular respiration relieves muscular fatigue, improves venous circulation, refreshes the body and mind, and increases mental energy. It also helps regulate the blood pressure, and cure psychosomatic complaints. We particularly recommend it to those suffering from overtiredness, insomnia or cardiac troubles.

Important Note

We shall now move on to the two simple Pranayama exercises, without retention of the breath, namely Ujjayi and Anuloma Viloma. These exercises are recommended to pregnant women by great exponents of Hathayoga. Ujjayi Pranayama is an excellent way of preparing the mother for childbirth; for while she practises, she learns, fairly, how to breathe in quickly but deeply and to regulate the amount of air she breathes out during long exhalations. We have used the technique of this Pranayama as the basis for two specifically designed breathing exercises for the period when the mother is pushing down and expelling the child (See pp.63-64). Regular and prolonged practice of Ujjayi and the other respiratory exercises contained in the present chapter are required for the pregnant woman to achieve the best results. Perfect control of the breath allows the mother fully to collaborate with the doctor and midwife during labour, and to deliver the newborn gently, with a minimum of fatigue and pain.

Ujjayi Pranayama
Breathing with Partial Closure of the Glottis

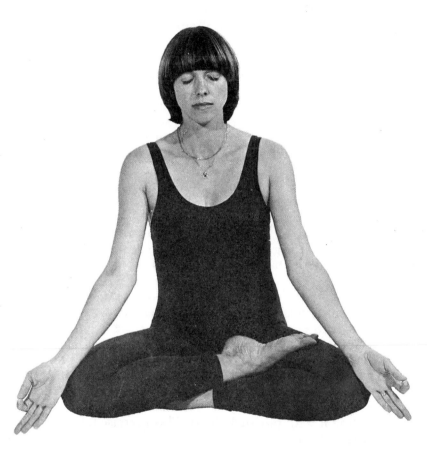

Fig. 81

Ujjayi Pranayama : Breathing with Partial Closure of the Glottis
Providing the mother-to-be has no respiratory problems, she may begin
practising this Pranayama from the very first lesson. The exercise involves half
or partial closure of the glottis by the slight contraction of the neck muscles,
thereby producing a low continuous sound, similar to a very soft snoring sound
throughout the Pranayama. It gives the impression of breathing through the
throat rather than the nose. The traditional method of performing the exercise

is to inhale through the two nostrils and exhale only through the left one. The authors prefer, however, to follow the advice of Swami Kuvalayananda[3] and teach pupils to practise this Pranayama by exhaling through both nostrils.

Sit cross-legged or in the Half-Lotus Posture, palms of the hands resting on the knees, or hands open, wrists resting on the knees, with the thumb and index finger forming a circle, and the other three fingers outstretched (Jnana-Mudra).

Having emptied the lungs, inhale on the three levels, i.e. abdominal, middle-chest and clavicular, at the same time expanding the rib cage as far as possible, as indicated for this Pranayama. Exhale, slightly contracting the abdominal muscles, until the chest shrinks to its smallest size and the lungs are empty.

Simple Pranayama, without retention of the breath, is practised in a 1:2 ratio, i.e. the duration of inhalation is always half that of exhalation. In the early stages, Pranayama may, for example, be performed at a rate of four seconds for breathing in and eight seconds for breathing out. At a later stage, it is possible to increase the duration, e.g. five seconds for inhalation and ten seconds for exhalation instead of four eight, providing this is comfortable.

Begin with five respirations a day, with four seconds inhalation and eight seconds exhalation for the first week, then subsequently increase the number of respirations by one or two a week, arriving at a maximum of twelve successive Ujjayi Pranayama respirations. Do not forget that one also has to perform the breathing exercises specifically designed for childbirth.

During this Pranayama, direct the attention to the flow of air and the pressure it will cause on the glottis, providing the neck muscles are contracted sufficiently. This gentle friction clears away the mucus and prevents coughing.

Ujjayi Pranayama produces a tonic effect on the nervous and glandular systems, as well as the digestive and eliminatory organs, such as pancreas, liver, stomach, intestines and kidneys. It develops the breathing capacity by rendering the chest more supple. Since good breathing depends on the elasticity of the lungs, even a few minutes' training in this Pranayama will help the lungs function better for the next 24 hours and thereby improve the oxygenation of the body during this period. The blood circulation also improves, thereby benefiting not only the mother but also the baby she is carrying by feeding it with purified blood. This exercise revitalises the brain and fosters better concentration.

In our course for pregnant women, we begin by taching complete *yogic* breathing, Ujjayi Pranayama and the specific exercises so that the future mother learns how to breathe correctly during pregnancy and childbirth. Once she has fully assimilated these exercises, at the right moment, she can pass on to Anuloma Viloma—i.e., breathing through alternate nostrils—which is without equal as far as the purification of the nerves is concerned.

---

3. The late Swami Kuvalayananda was the founder and head of the Kaivalyadhama Yogic Health Institute, Lonavla, India.

Ujjayi and Anuloma Viloma can be practised one after the other, but the number of repetitions must be reduced, otherwise the lungs will become tired. When performed properly, the *Pranayama* exercises tend to strengthen the lungs and accumulate reserves of *prana*—vital energy. If practised one after the other, Anuloma Viloma should come before Ujjayi.

Anuloma Viloma

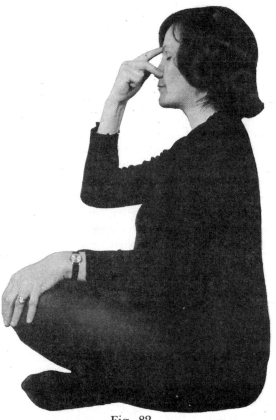

Fig. 82

Anuloma Viloma

Sit cross-legged, with the left hand resting on the left knee. With the thumb and third finger of the right hand, close alternate nostrils. For the sake of convenience, the index finger is placed between the eyebrows. Empty the lungs, and begin by inhaling through the left nostril and exhaling through the right one, then inhale through the right nostril and exhale through the left one. This represents one complete alternate respiration. We recommend allowing four seconds for inhalation and eight for exhalation. The Pranayama should be practised three to seven times per session. Begin with three respirations, and increase the number by one or two a week, practising every day. Direct the concentration to the flow of air through each respective nostril.

The physical effects of this exercise help improve the oxygenation of the blood, and bring the metabolism and hormonal secretions into balance. The Pranayama is recommended for curing certain kinds of headache, and in particular, for purifying the nerves—nadis. The psychic effects help develop the concentration, foster clear thinking and provide calm and serenity to mind and body. Having practised Pranayama, we finish the course by helping mothers to prepare mentally for childbirth.

Mental Preparation For Childbirth

Childbirth is one of the outstanding events in the life of a woman. The self-control she must exercise in order to overcome her apprehension and the pain caused by labour and the birth of her child, help her to develop on a psychological plane and turn her into a more mature person.

The pain experienced during childbirth is natural and has nothing to do with illness. In any case, it disappears without trace as soon as the child is born. If the future mother prepares for childbirth feeling calm, confident and brave, the event will take place with a minimum of pain and energy. According to Yoga, a woman's mental attitude towards childbirth is as important as the event itself. The mother should ensure that she maintains a positive mental outlook throughout her pregnancy, in order to influence favourable development of embryo and to prepare herself for giving birth to a healthy, happy child. How can this positive attitude be achieved?

The physical exercises the mother practises for a few moments every day are not enough to achieve the desired results. Since Yoga is a way of life which favours the quest for harmony and inner peace, the future mother should lead a healthy, well-balanced existence in which she practises control of the mind and tries to think only constructive thoughts. As the gardener keeps his garden in order by removing the weeds which spring up in it, so the pregnant woman should learn the art of 'gardening' her mind, i.e. weeding out the negative thoughts in favour of the positive ones. In this way, for example, an unselfish thought will immediately neutralise a selfish one.

Those who allow only positive thoughts into their mind and who practise the art of thwarting negative ones will live in harmony and advance rapidly along the road of self-perfection. Positive autosuggestion is a particularly effective means of achieving this end.

Those who constantly suggest powerful, patient and hopeful ideas to themselves, even when external circumstances are not always favourable to this; who refuse to let themselves give in to discouragement; and who persistently maintain a confident outlook through autosuggestion will attain a considerable degree of self-control.

110

To be truly effective, the asanas must also be accompanied by autosuggestion. During Savasana, the Dead Pose, which is also named the Posture of Complete yogic Relaxation, by suggesting to oneself "I am calm and relaxed", one feels completely relaxed. During other asanas, one directs the attention towards the various organs which the asanas are designed to regenerate, such as the thyroid or the solar plexus.

By way of example, let us take the case of Sarvangasana, named the Shoulder Stand. It has a revitalising effect on the thyroid gland, and, through this gland, on the entire organism. While practising this inverted posture, because of the position of the head and neck, one feels an influx of fresh blood regenerating the neck region, towards which one's attention has to be directed. By suggesting to oneself that the thyroid gland is functioning better, one will considerably increase the beneficial effects of this asana.

Autosuggestion strengthens to a maximum the regenerative power of the Hathayoga exercises.

> *"Autosuggestion is the greatest energy of all, and it is the greatest of all cures. By it, a man can alleviate, minimize, eliminate fear of pain (...), fear of suffering, mental conflicts, and may obtain freedom and liberation from all bondages."*

B. KRISHNAYYA

Through the control of her thoughts and emotions, and through autosuggestion combined with specific physical exercises and, more especially, breathing control, the future mother stands a good chance of overcoming the difficulties she may possibly encounter during childbirth, thus successfully and fearlessly bringing a child into the world while remaining in control of the situation. We shall now turn to the practical aspect of this discipline.

Concentration on the Words of the Yogis and Sages

The future mother sits cross-legged and closes her eyes. She then begins to meditate on a specific thought, such as:

> *"Our happiness or our unhappiness, our force or our weakness, our progress or regression always depend on our attitude, our way of understanding things and people, and the way we react to them."*
>
> *"The belief in success stimulates our efforts."*
>
> *"Our personal development is influenced by each of our thoughts and deeds."*
>
> *"We become what we think, and reap what we sow."*

DHAMMAPADA

Having spent a few moments relaxing, we move on to the final exercise in preparation for childbirth.

Autosuggestion

Adopt a sitting position, legs crossed and back straight. Close the eyes and withdraw the mind from the outside world. Direct the mind within oneself, towards the breathing. Breathe slowly, deeply and regularly according to complete Yogic breathing. Tell yourself that with each inhalation, you are filling the body with prana, the cosmic energy contained in the air, and that with each exhalation, while expelling impure air you are assimilating the life-giving energy just inhaled, allowing it to penetrate every fibre of your being. Think of the body as being healthy and of the mind as being strong, and that the child one is carrying is developing normally.

Autosuggestion

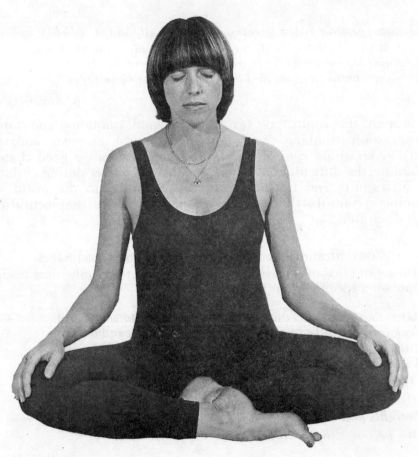

Fig. 83

Say to oneself that every thing will turn out fine.....

The future mother should mentally prepare her childbirth by visualising it, living through it in her thoughts, and picturing to herself what its various stages will be like. She should banish all fear from her mind, and remain confident, calm and serene. Thus she will approach the moment of birth in the best possible conditions.

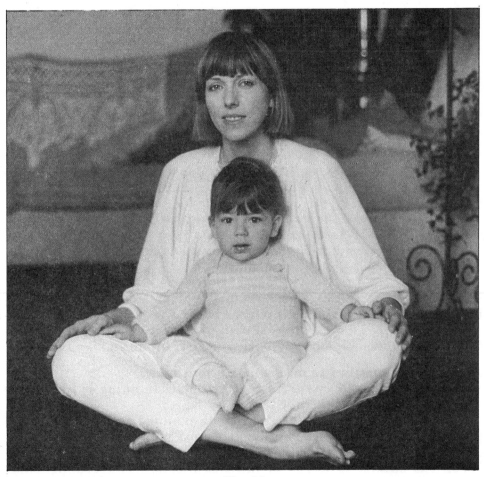

Fig. 84

..... and that the baby will be sound in body and mind, with all the physical and moral qualities one would like him to possess.

Morning and Evening Exercises to be Practised at Home Before Breakfast and Dinner

Since our course takes place only once or twice a week, we advise pregnant women to practise daily in their own home the exercises they have learned on the course.

Important Note

The instructions received during the course must be followed very strictly. Depending on the future mother's state of health and the stage of pregnancy, some exercises are highly recommended while others should be avoided. A choice of several exercises is offered, to be practised in the *morning on rising,* which do not last long.

(1) Sit cross-legged and perform several complete Yogic respirations This helps oxygenate the body and creates a feeling of well-being throughout the rest of the day.

(2) Begin with Modified Paschimottanasana (See Fig. 48) or Modified Janusirasana (See Fig. 49).

(3) Move on to *Modified Ardha-Matsyendrasana* or *Modified Vakrasana* (See. Fig. 59).

(4) Next comes Catuspadasana (See Fig. 62)
The combination of these four *asanas* prevents back pains and tones the spinal column.

(5) At this point, relax for a moment, feet raised and against the wall, then continue with Modified Viparita Karani (See Fig. 74) or Modified Sarvangasana (See Fig. 76).
These exercises irrigate the brain, revitalise the nervous and glandular system, and are very effective for those lacking sleep.

(6) Bring the exercises to an end with Matsyasana (See Fig. 77), then spend a few moments relaxing while lying on one side.

(7) Now pass on to Ujjayi Pranayama (See Fig. 81) and, depending on instructions received during the course, add Anuloma Viloma ((See Fig. 82). If the latter is added, it should be practised before Ujjay.

These two breathing exercises purify the nerves, ensure the correct functioning of the hormones, and make one feel strong and healthy.

Exercises to be practised in the evening, before dinner

Starting with relaxation on either side Chapter 9 and finishing with Ustrasana and the posture for relaxing the back (See Fig. 57).

Choose one of the three back-stretching postures, and one meditation posture. Eliminate Modified Paschimottanasana and Modified Janusirasana if these have already been performed during the morning session. On the other hand, it is possible to repeat one inverted posture in the evening: either Modified Viparita Karani or Modified Sarvangasana.

Those who are particularly active and fit can choose one or two of the seven asanas mentioned in pp. 87-94, and practise them either in the morning or evening, combined with the other postures.

Once the series of exercises is over, perform complete Yogic relaxation (See p.104) and finish off by mental preparation for childbirth (See pp. 103-104)

The different kinds of relaxation either lying on the back, on the side, feet against the the wall, or kneeling, head and trunk bent forwards—can be repeated two or three times a day, if one feels the need for them. Should one wish, it is possible to perform all the exercises recommended during the course, in a single session, either in the morning or evening.

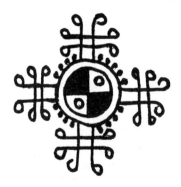

Harmony of Body and Mind

"If the food which the mother takes in its assimilated form goes into the production of the body and form of the child in her womb, then to a great extent the thoughts of the mother during her pregnancy give a direction and an impetus to the psychological make-up of the child.[1]" Each of our thoughts and emotions does indeed create repercussions on the cells of the body and leaves its mark on them. "The thoughts expressed by a pregnant woman, the emotions which make her heart beat, and the words she utters, produce a strong vibration in each cell of her body and leave their deep imprint on her inner psychological constitution." These vibrations are felt by the baby inside her. Today, it is a well-known fact that many children born of a mother who underwent a deep emotional shock or who experienced great fear during pregnancy can show signs of nervous deficiency.

So just as the food absorbed and assimilated by the future mother allows the child she is carrying to develop physically, the thoughts she has during pregnancy will produce an effect on the child's mental development.

To take an example, it is highly unadvisable for pregnant women to watch films depicting scenes of horror, murder, violence or pornography, for these can produce a negative effect on the future child's character.

In country areas, care is always taken to ensure that a mother-to-be never enters the presence of a seriously wounded person. A story is told that a pregnant woman who saw her husband accidentally cut his hand off with a scythe gave birth to a one-handed child.

One of the authors' own ancestors is said to have been so impressed by a novel in which the heroine had a lock of white in her otherwise dark hair that she gave birth to a girl with the same unusual colouring.

In very ancient Hindu Scriptures, such as the *Puranas* and *Upanishads*, there are numerous references to prenatal education and to the fact that the child hears and reacts to sounds and voices outside, all of which has been confirmed by modern medicine.

---

1. "Discourses on *Aitreya Upanishad*", Swami Chinmayananda.

It is said that if a pregnant woman constantly meditates on a *Rishi*, Great Sage, whose picture she has in front of her, and reflects on all his virtues, her child will resemble the model which has inspired her.

In the *Mahabharata*, we hear how Arjuna's wife, listening daily to the tales of battle told by her husband, ardently desired to conceive a child similar to the warriors in the stories. In the end, she gave birth to the hero, Virabhimanyu, who knew all the secrets of the art of war without ever having had to learn them. While still in the womb, Virabhimanyu had in fact overheard his father revealing the secrets to his mother, which is why he was an invincible hero from early youth onwards.

An ancient Hindu legend relates an interesting incident concerning the influence of thoughts of the mother and the atmosphere around her can produce on the child she is carrying.

There was once in India a cruel and wicked king who reigned by terror and who was surrounded by evil courtiers. His wife became pregnant, and shortly after, the king went into the forest in order to do penance, thereby to increase his dominion and occult powers.

Having learned of the queen's condition, through divine inspiration, a great Sage came to visit her at the palace and suggested that she should escape from the harmful influence of those surrounding her. The queen followed the Rishi's advice and agreed to accompany him to his *Ashram*, a place of religious retreat, where she stayed until the end of her pregnancy.

At the Ashram, she spent several months in a peaceful, religious atmosphere. The Sage made her follow a purification discipline, and explained the holy Scriptures to her. The young queen practised Yoga, meditated, and prayed to God that the child, she was carrying would become imbued with all the learning she was herself acquiring. She asked Heaven to send her a child full of wisdom and virtue, strong enough to thwart the fiendish plots of her husband, the king, and able to help suffering mankind.

When the time came, the queen returned to the palace and gave birth to a prince. Having learned of the birth, the kind also returned to the palace, but with the intention of bringing the prince up according to his own wicked principles. All the raja's attempts to influence and corrupt his son proved vain, however, for the young prince had been so deeply affected by his mother's pious thoughts and the atmosphere reigning in the Ashram at which she had stayed while carrying him, that he subsequently became an exemplary monarch, a model of goodness, purity, wisdom and piety, who devoted his life to the hapiness of his people.

From this we can see that whatever the circumstances, the future mother should try to lead a peaceful, well-balanced life, and avoid all negative feelings, such as anger, jealousy, hate, desire for vengeance, etc. Every morning, she should wake up thinking of the well-being of every living thing. Her husband should help preserve a harmonious atmosphere at home, making sure he protects and safeguards his wife.

During pregnancy, she should keep company only with people who have a favourable influence over her. She should read fine literature, look at beautiful works of art, listen to soft music, contemplate pleasant landscapes, and have only positive, constructive thoughts.

These will engender favourable currents, not only for the future mother's health, but also for her peace of mind. In this way, the tiny being she is carrying inside her will be filled with beauty and harmony, and will show good physical, mental and spiritual development.

"Health is the highest gain,
Contentment is the greatest wealth (...),
Nibbana (peace) is the bliss supreme.

BUDDHA

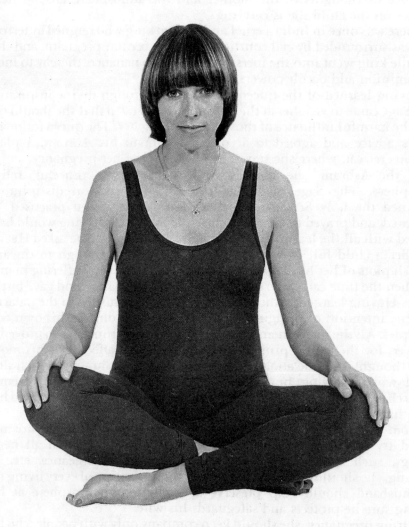

Fig. 85

118

Diet During Pregnancy

One should eat little but often.

AYURVEDA

The pregnant woman should eat little but often, at regular hours, through-out the day, rather than consuming large quantities of food at mealtimes. Since it is she who is supporting the child growing inside her, she requires a highly balanced diet, which must be prolonged after childbirth into the weaning period. The future mother must avoid over-eating. Moderation is the rule prescribed by the thousand-year-old medical science of Ayurveda. *One should only eat when one is genuinely hungry, and leave the table without feeling bloated.*

The mother-to-be should eat healthy, natural food—preferably untreated—and avoid food which is overcooked or contains too much fat, sugar or seasoning. It is better to avoid meat—especially red meat, or consume very little, for meat engenders toxins in the organism. On the other hand, fish can be recommended, because it is rich in minerals. Non-vegetarians suffering from iron defficiency can eat liver and kidneys.

Vegetarianism is a common practice in India, and many people have come to us for advice concerning the foodstuffs which contain the most proteins. We should like to reply here by indicating the foodstuffs which are richest in vegetable proteins, as well as other products vital to the health, on account of the fact that they contain minerals and vitamins.

It is important to eat cereals: wheat, maize, oats, rye, rice, wholemeal bread, wholemeal flower, and dry vegetables: lentils, dhal, dried peas, chickpeas, beans, soya—beans or beansprouts, and tapioca containing protein.

We recommend eating dairy products: milk (a complete food), curd and cottage cheese rich in calcium.

Fresh fruit and vegetables are rich in vitamins and indispensable to a balanced vegetarian diet. Spinach, lettuce, potatoes, celery and artichoke hearts, apples, bananas, and papaya contain large quantities of iron. Juicy fruits—lemons, oranges, pineapple, papaya, apples, all green vegetables, soya and nuts contain calcium.

Magnesium is contained in regular vegetables, other vegetables with green leaves, different varieties of nuts, and non-refined cereals.

Potassium is contained in treacle, whole grains, and almonds.

Not to be forgotten are honey, non-refined sugar, figs and dates, which all provide instant energy.[1]

Those suffering from constipation are advised to eat apples. grapes, stewed prunes and figs and thin vegetable soup. One should not eat fruit or drink fruit juice after cheese. because this leads to fermentation within the digestive system and provokes flatulence.

Whether or not she follows a vegetarian diet, the future mother needs to absorb proteins, calcium, iron and mineral salts, which make it possible for the skeleton and muscular tissue of the embryo to form. She should take vitamins A, B, C, D and E, for these are indispensable. They are contained in the foodstuffs recommended above.

Alcohol and tobacco are forbidden during pregnancy, and the consumption of tea and coffee should be reduced.

Sample Menus for a Single Day [2]

Studies have shown that a person's energy during the day is to a large extent due to what he has eaten for breakfast. This meal should therefore be nourishing and ensure the body an adequate supply of proteins and carbohydrates such as honey, treacle, cane sugar, maize, puffed rice, etc.

Breakfast

On rising, it is possible to eat a piece of fruit or drink some unchilled fruit juice. Breakfast consists of a cup of tea or coffee with milk, or plain milk or Ovaltine, and cereals: porridge, cornflakes, a slice of wholemeal bread or *Ryvita*, wholemeal biscuits, *Dar Vida* or wholemeal cakes with honey—a maximum of one soupspoon per day to avoid gaining weight and butter. If desired, one or two soft-boiled eggs can replace the cereals.

Lunch

Vegetarians can begin the meal with raw vegetables, followed by a choice of lentils, dhal, various kinds of beans, chickpeas or soya, all of which are rich in proteins. They can also eat fresh vegetables of the season, e.g. aubergine curry (see. p. 158), peas and mushrooms (see. p. 158) with rice, green salad, curd or cottage cheese. The meal is rounded off by a dessert such as pudding or stewed fruit, or fruit salad.

Teatime

Teatime consists of not-too strong tea with milk or lemon, milk on its own (or mixed with syrup or Ovaltine), or fresh fruit juice. We suggest eating a slice of wholemeal bread, gingerbread, or one or two wholemeal cakes with butter and a little honey.

---

1. Cf. *Yoga, Harmony of Body and Mind*, Chapter VI, "A Well-Balanced Diet".
2. Several vegetarian recipes using the foodstuffs described in this section are included at the back of the book.

Dalia in Dinner

This meal begins with mixed salad or vegetable soup, followed by a dish of cereals: wheat semolina, Dalia in Indian parlance, wheat couscous, a North African dish, an Italian pasta, wheat pilpil boulghour or polenta, according to choice, plus fresh vegetables. Those who like rice may eat pullao with almonds or lemon rice (See. p. 155).

For dessert, one may eat curd, fresh or dried fruit, carrot halva or coconut cake (See. p.159). One can also make a Swiss country dinner consisting of boiled potatoes in their jackets with butter and cheese—gruyere, fribourg, or processed cheese—and mixed salad.

To take another example, we recommend eating Bircher Muesli (See. p. 159). with wholemeal bread and butter, accompanied bby herbal tea. At bedtime, one may drink a coup of milk with saffron or milk with honey. It is also possible to drink a camomile tea with a slice of lemon, lime-blossom tea, verbena tea, etc., with honey or unrefined sugar.

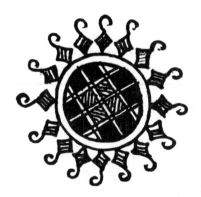

The Childbirth

Many women, especially those who are pregnant for the first time ask us what they should do at moment of birth. They are often apprehensive about this event because they think that there is a chance of dying while giving birth, and whatever happens, childbirth causes the mother great physical pain. In fact, one should begin by telling oneself that giving birth is one of the most natural things in the world, and that the practice of *Yoga* helps the future mother to overcome her fear and prepare her effectively for the event.

When the moment comes for giving birth, the woman needs to feel protected, well taken care-of and surrounded by loving affection. The pains felt during labour often stem from the fact that the mothers resistance is the result of her inability to rationalise how completely to relax and let herself go. Breathing plays a crucial role in helping to push the baby out of her body.

In Ancient India, three positions were recommended for childbirth:
1) standing, knees spread and slightly bent;
2) squatting ; and
3) lying on the back, legs bent, the trunk, knees and feet spread apart. This position of lying on the back is one of the most commonly used postures today.

Women often ask whether pushing down on the baby to expel it requires a great effort. Yoga teaches us, however, how to relax the body, so is the answer to let oneself go and allow the baby to be born without strain. The mother should avoid resistance, fear and irritation, for allowing everything to happen calmly and serenely.

A woman who is tense and on edge will feel pain because she is resisting and thereby hindering the child from emerging. Such a state of mind as this leads to genital tension and causes suffering by blocking the smooth, painless birth of the infant.

The practice of Yoga develops the ability to relax once the contractions begin, stills the future mother's fears, and helps her learn the required patience and calm so that she can co-operate more effectively at the moment of birth.

The mother should not try to find ways from what appears to be pain, but simply confront and accept it. This is the only way through which she can free herself from fear and suffering. Through autosuggestion, she will be able to overcome this fear, and thus bravely face and accept the act of giving birth. The more confidence and self-control she possesses, the less pain she will feel.

Everything should be ready for the baby's arrival some two weeks before the child is due. The future mother should prepare the things she will need for herself and the baby during maternity.

She should be admitted to hospital as soon as the contractions become more frequent and regular, preferably before the mother starts losing liquids. She should opt for natural childbirth and, choose to remain conscious throughout the act of bringing her baby into the world—this means saying no to drugs and anaesthetics. Childbirth normally takes place in three stages:

    1. Dilatation

    2. Expulsion—1 & 2 together are known as labour

    3. Delivery.

1. Dilatation or Opening-Up

Lasting up to 20 hours, this is the stage where the mouth of the uterus opens fully so that it can accommodate the head of the foetus and allow the baby to pass down the genital canal at the moment of birth. The mouth of the uterus dilates as a result of the contractions of the uterine muscles. The contractions gives one a feeling of a tugging sensation in the lumbar region; at a later stage, they push the baby downwards in order to expel it.

To begin with, these involuntary, intermittent and rhythmic contractions take place roughly at the interval of every 20 minutes. The frequency increases and by the end of the opening-up period, they occur every five minutes, and then every two or three minutes. As they grow more frequent, they last longer.

Many women fear the pain these contractions can cause. Yoga remedies this by constituting a discipline which teaches mother-to-be how to remain calm and self-controlled, and how to relax and breathe correctly during the different stages of childbirth.

At the beginning of the opening-up period, when the contractions are infrequent and not very strong, the mother should relax, while at the same time practising deep breathing on the three levels, i.e. complete yogic breathing.

Between contractions, she should try to continue breathing deeply and regularly; for on a physical level, this will ensure the oxygenation required for herself and the baby.

This technique of deep rhythmic breathing ensures a harmonious functioning of the whole system including the brain, and helps, on a psychological level, to calm the emotions and create a feeling of well-being. To achieve this, the future mother should, whenever possible, take a few moments to collect her thoughts. She should make herself comfortable, close her eyes and retire within herself, thereby creating a sense of inner calm and serenity, just as she has learned during the Yoga course in the exercises designed to prepare her mentally for childbrith.

During the period of dilatation, she should have thoughts of a positive kind—i.e. endurance, patience and confidence. It would be of great help if her husband were present. The mother needs to know that she can rely on his help and encouragement. He can aid her to relax and retire within herself.

When the contractions continue for a longer period and become more frequent, she should avoid abdominal breathing, and simply perform middle-chest and clavicular breathing (See Chapter 9 'Complete Yogic Breathing', and p. 62, 'the Different Methods of Specific Respiration').

In India, a remedy for soothing the pains, caused by the contractions, is gently to massage the mother's coccyx—i.e. tip of the spinal column with small triangular bone—with almond or sesame oil, or to apply warm compresses to the lower back.

The future mother should approach the period of strong contractions in a positive way. By continuing to practise autosuggestion, she will be able to remove all fear of pain, all uneasiness, and this will enable her to remain calm and relaxed. The more she is able to control her emotions and maintain psychic balance, the less pain she will feel during childbirth.

2. Expulsion

The transition between the full opening of the mouth of the uterus and the birth of the baby is known as expulsion. It lasts some ten to twenty minutes, but can be longer or shorter. In the case of a first child, it usually takes the mother longer to give birth. Those who have followed a preparation course will find, however, that birth takes place more easily and quickly.

Throughout the period of expulsion, the mother should push during contractions and relax between them, in order to muster her energy for when she next pushes. At this point, having exhaled, she should inhale deeply, and with full lungs and a closed mouth and glottis, contract the abdominal muscles and push. Exhalation through the mouth should sound like a sigh of relief "Ha. a.a.a..." (See Exercise 1,   p. 63).

An effective way of continuing to push is to exhale slowly through the nose, making sure the glottis is partly closed. The mother should push against her breath when contracting the abdominal muscles and lowering the diaphragm (See Exercise 2,   p.64)

This way of adjusting the glottis is taught during the Yoga course while practising Ujjayi Pranayama. It enables the mother to regulate the amount of air she exhales and to push longer without becoming out of breath or using up energy in vain. As she lets out the breath through the nose, she emits a low, continuous sound.

When the head is expelled, the mother should inhale and exhale, deeply and regularly performing middle and upper-chest respiration (without abdominal breathing). Following the instructions of the doctor or midwife, the mother should then resume pushing slightly, so that the rest of the child's body slips out, and the baby is born.

In India, astrologers establish a child's birth chart from the moment he takes his breath and utters his first cry, for it is only once the child has begun to breathe that he is truly alive: *"Breath is life"*.

Within five minutes following the birth of the child, the umbilical chord leading from his abdomen and connected to the placenta should be ligatured and severed, but only after it has stopped pulsating.

3. Delivery

Once the baby has been born, the mother continues to experience a series of contractions, sometimes barely perceptible, which prepare for the expulsion of the placenta. This is expelled some 20 to 30 minutes after the child is born. The placenta is the organ through which oxygen and nutritional substances are absorbed by the embryo. It also stores vitamins and manufactures hormones. The placenta links the embryo to the maternal uterus during pregnancy. While still inside the mother, the foetus floats in the 'waters' of the amnion—a membrane enveloping the child within the womb i.e. uterus.

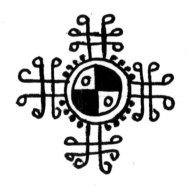

Post-Natal Care of the Mother

During the five or six weeks following childbirth, the mother requires special post-natal care. It is advisable for her to stay at home for some ten days in order to rest and allow her genital organs to return to their usual position. Often the uterus is overweight after childbirth, but is subsequently returns to normal. To begin with, it can sometimes lack elasticity as well.

As of the third or fourth week, the mother can attend to household tasks without feeling fatigued, but should avoid carrying heavy weights, climbing too many stairs, or travelling by motorcar.

Some women still feel pain three or four days after childbirth. Their breasts may hurt once they begin breast-feeding their child, and this can have repercussions on the uterus. Abdominal bandages may be used because they not only make the woman feel that she is comfortable, but support the abdominal wall while at the same time exerting slight pressure on the womb.

The mother should wear a bra, preferably cotton, to support the breasts from crushing. The child should suck at the mother's breast, since this helps the milk to rise. The nipples will swell and harden due to the influx of liquid. During the lactation period, the mother should take special care of her breasts. It is important for her thoroughly to wash the nipples in boiled water both before and after each breat-feeding session. Having done this, she can smear a little oil or cream on the nipples to prevent painful fissures.

Should the mother suffer from breast fissures, sores or irritations, we recommend that she wash the breasts in a camomile, (flower) an aromatic solution. Put 12 heads of camomile in ¾ litre of Evian mineral water. Boil for four to five minutes, then drain off the solution obtained. This preparation can be used for several washes in a single day, but only the quantity required for each respective wash need be heated in a saucepan. Apply the solution using a light lukewarm compress on the breasts, such as absorbent cotton soaked in the solution. Having thoroughly patted (and not rubbed) them dry, very gently massage the breasts with a pommade, cream bottled French spring water. If not available, use any pure spring or well water recommended by the doctor (e.g. Ceratum) available at the chemist's, and cover them with a compress of soft gauze.

In India, the Yogis state that the best foodstuffs for a breast-feeding mother are cereals, vegetables, fruit and dairy products, with water and milk to drink

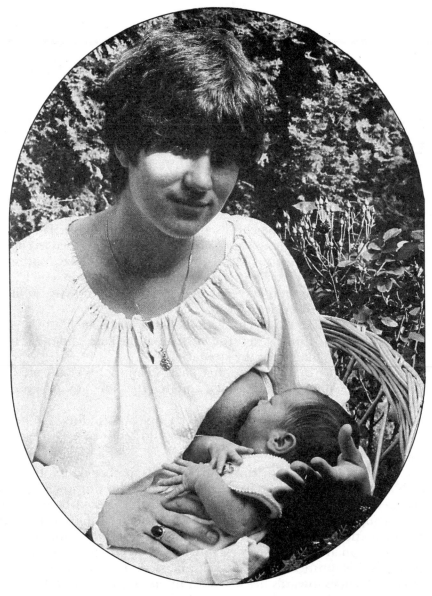

Fig. 86

127

Care of the Newborn

Having cut the umbilical chord and made sure that the knot has been correctly tied, one should attend to the infant's eyes by washing them in water containing boric acid and inserting two drops of fresh silver-nitrate lotion.

In India, once the newborn child has been washed, it is rubbed with oil and dried in a soft towel. The abdominal region and navel should be cleansed with alcohol or other disinfectant. A sterile dressing should be applied to the navel before one surrounds the child's abdomen with an elastic bandage. Its clothes should be light and loose, and should not be so tight so as to constrict or restrain its free movement. The baby's cradle should be comfortably equipped with a tiny matress. The head should rest in a position which allows him to breathe normally and correctly and to eliminate mucus the mouth should be wiped off with a clean cloth.

It is good for the child to lie on his back, but after meals he should be placed on his side. To enable him to exert the muscles of the back and neck, he can from time to time be placed on the stomach.

It is vital to ensure that the hot water bags warming his cradle are firmly closed and do not contain boiling water, and that the baby's room is properly ventilated.

The infant should be washed with each change of swaddling-clothes, and once the navel wound has closed, he or she should be given a bath every day.

The Newborn Child's Diet

The best nourishment the baby can be given is his mother's milk. It provides him with all the things he needs in order to grow and immunises him against certain illnesses. The mother's milk is not only easily digested, but is always at the correct temperature. The mortality rate for breast-fed infants is lower than the rate for bottle-fed babies. On a psychological level, the child feels more secure. The intimate relationship established between child and mother is indeed vital to his future balance and happiness. As for the mother, she feels protective and tender towards her newborn infant when she sees the pleasure and joy he takes in being fed at her breast.

Some women are reluctant to breast-feed their child because it may possibly take too long. They should not forget, however, that preparing a baby's bottle is also a time-consuming process. Others fear that their breasts will become mis-shapen. They need have no qualms, however, for breast—feeding will not distort or harm the breasts—quite the contrary, it is an excellent remedy for breasts distended by pregnancy. The father should encourage the mother to breast-feed their child.

According to *Ayurveda*, another excellent substance is honey. In India, a tiny quantity is gently applied to the newborn's tongue. Later on, the daily amount can be increased to one teaspoon a day, given in two separate doses. Until the fourth month, however, the child should only be fed with milk.

As of the fifth month, the baby should gradually be weaned onto other easily assimilated foods, i.e. thin soups, stewed fruit, curd, purees and fruit juices. Nor should one forget to give him small but sufficient quantities of water to drink.

It is imperative to avoid overfeeding the child : Mothers should make sure that his diet does not contain too much sugar or fatty food. A plump child is never healthy, and has a low resistance to disease.

Later on, care must be taken to ensure that the youngster does not eat too many sweets or drink too many sugary beverages.

Breast-Feed is Best

What is love?
Love knows no bargaining,
Love knows no fear,
Love is always for love's sake.

Swami Vivekananda

In order to develop in harmonious surroundings, a child needs the love and care of his parents.

In recent years, more emphasis has been laid than in the past on the fact that both the mother and the father should if possible take personal care of their child. It has been discovered that children lacking in affection or proper attention from their parents tend to waste away and later experience difficulty in adjustment; in some cases, they do become maladjusted.

Nature has endowed the mother with the ability to feed her child at the breast. There can be no doubt that babies either fed in this way or bottle-fed while being lovingly held in the arms grow faster. The child needs physical contact in order to grow. From the moment he is born, he requires this reassuring and pleasure-giving contact, constituting an initial experience which will produce long-lasting effects.

A child brought up in an atmosphere of love and understanding by parents who wish to see him grow into a happy, confident and lively person, will enjoy good relations with others throughout his entire life. On the other hand, a child who is not brought up in the conditions required for him to develop harmoniously—due to lack of love from parents who do not devote enough time to him—will become distrustful and hostile towards others.

Scientists and educators, all agree that a child deprived of affection and tender care during his earliest infancy will suffer the effects of this throughout his life and will be unable either physically or morally to attain full happiness.

One Example Among Many

During World War II, 45 babies were placed in a children's home, but there were only six nurses to look after them. Although the babies were given more food and medical attention than most children from poor backgrounds, they were deprived of warm, affectionate contact. The results were most alarming : the children showed signs of growth troubles, and were underdeveloped both physically and mentally. Some of them even went into a form of nervous depression, marked by a fixed, expressionless stare.

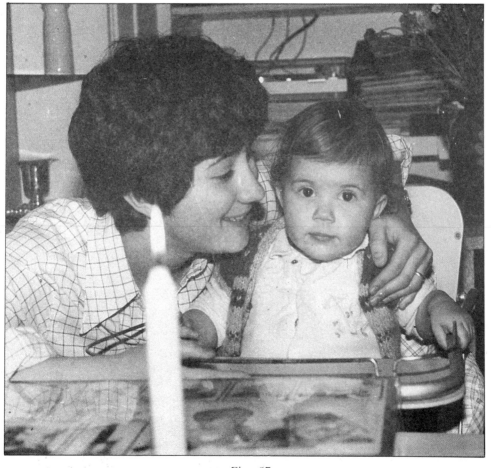

Fig. 87

Several of the children died, in spite of all the medical attention given to them, as if too apathetic even to go on living. Many cases of schizophrenia are also thought to originate from lack of love. To take a case the condition of a baby girl suffering from this illness was considerably improved as a result of the constant affection shown to her by the nurse at the hospital where she was being treated. Later on, she was even able to lead a normal married life.

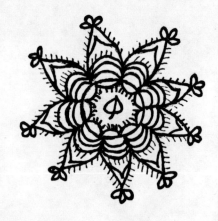

Regain Your Shape:
Exercises After Childbirth

The very next day after a normal childbirth, the mother can practise Catuspadasana—Cat Posture on All Fours, of (Fig. 62) to help her organs resume their normal position. Six weeks later, she can perform this exercise, pulling in the abdominal wall while completely contracting the abdominal muscles as she breathes out with the back hunched and the head lowered.

Providing she has not undergone episiotomy or experienced other complications, the mother can perform Asvini-Mudra in the Januvaksasana—symbol of the Mare in the Knee-Chest posture (Fig. 50) ten days after childbirth. Like the Cat Posture, this exercise helps the womb return to its proper position. It also restores to the muscles of the vagina, distended by childbirth, their original elasticity. Asvini-Mudra plays a role which is just as important after as during pregnancy. Since the exercise consists in alternately contracting and relaxing the muscles of the perineum and the entire pelvic region, it helps, first, to exercise and to relax to a maximum the vaginal muscles at the moment the baby is born and, second, to restore the muscle-tone once birth has taken place.

As of the sixth week, the mother can gradually resume practice of the other Hathayoga exercises. The following asanas are designed to strengthen the abdominal muscles, loosened by pregnancy, but a choice of exercise should be made according to one's individual abilities.

Asanas marked with an asterisk (*) should not be performed during menstruation.

Ardha-Halasana *
The Half Plough Posture

We recommend that one should begin the training of the abdominal muscles with this exercise, raising only one leg at a time. (Fig. 54) Repeat the exercise two or three times on either side.

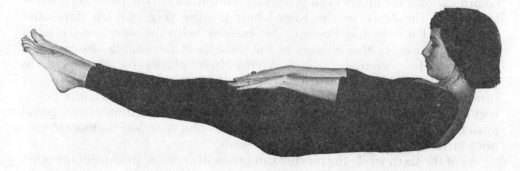

Fig. 88

Utthitapada-Merudandasana* : The Spinal-Column Posture, Legs Raised

Lie on the back, and place the hands on the thighs. Breathe in deeply, raise the head by bringing the chin close to the sternum, then raise the trunk and legs while keeping the feet some 30 cms off the ground. Stay in this position for five seconds, lungs full, directing the attention towards the abdominal region. Breathe out while at the same time resuming the original lying position, and relax.

This exercise can be practised 2 to 4 times in succession, gradually increasing the number of repetitions.

134

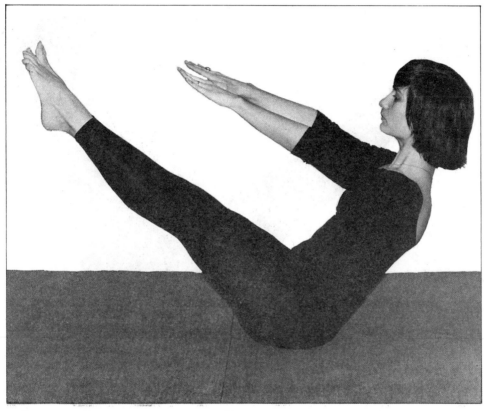

Fig. 89

Paripurna-Navasana* : The Boat Posture
Lie on the back, and while inhaling, raise the arms above the head. Exhale, at
the same time raising the head, trunk and legs. Hold the arms outstretched so
that they form a line parallel to the legs. Remain in this posture for a few
seconds, lungs empty, back straight, then taking a deep breath, resume the
lying position and relax. This exercise requires careful concentration if one is
to keep one's balance. It can be repeated two or three times.

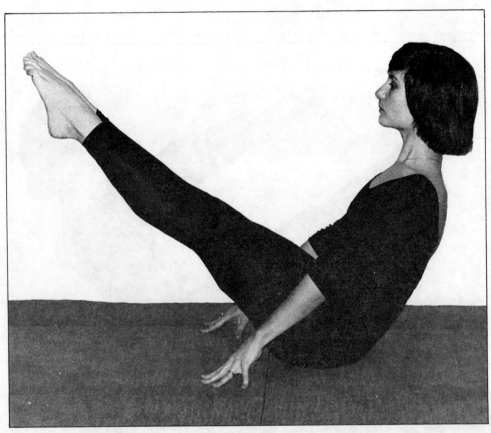

Fig. 90

Boat Posture, Hands on Ground* : Variation.
Sit with the legs outstretched, hands on the ground beside the top of the thighs.
Slightly tilt the trunk backwards. While breathing in deeply and maintaining
one's balance with the hands, slowly raise the legs some 60 cms off the ground.
Hold the posture for several seconds with lungs full; then gradually lower the
legs at the same speed, while exhaling, and relax. The attention should be
directed towards the abdominal region. Women who experience difficulty in
retaining the breath should breathe normally during the exercise. The asana
can be repeated two to three times in succession.

136

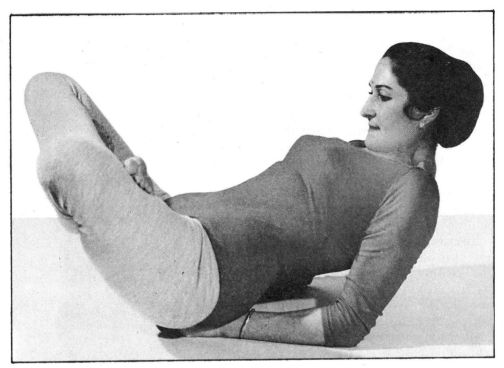

Fig. 91

Tolangulasana* : The Balance Posture

Position the legs as if for the Lotus posture, Padmasana, then tilt the trunk backwards, supporting the body with the elbows. Clench the hands and place them beneath the buttocks. Using the clenched hands and the forearms as a lever, bring the head forwards, and raise the trunk and legs so that the abdominal muscles are fully contracted.

In order to increase intra-abdominal pressure, thereby toning the internal organs, breathe in deeply before raising the trunk and legs, and retain the posture for a few seconds, lungs full. Direct the attention towards the abdominal region. Relax in a sitting position.

This asana is particularly recommended for restoring the stomach distended by pregnancy to its original shape. It is also an effective way of ensuring muscles tone. The exercise should not be performed by those with abnormal blood pressure, a weak heart or lungs, or by those suffering from ulcers.

It can be performed two or three times in succession.

Yoga-Mudra With Stretching of Back and Arms*

Sit in the Lotus position Cross the fingers and, while turning the palms of the hands upwards, raise the arms above the head. While breathing in, stretch the arms and back, remain two seconds in this position, with lungs full, and then breathe out slowly leaning the trunk forwards until, with the open palms turned outwards, the thumbs are touching the ground. Rest the forehead on the ground and remain in this stretched posture with the back straight for five seconds. Remember to draw in and contract the abdominal muscles while performing this posture.

Inhale deeply while raising the trunk and arms, then stretch once again before lowering the hands and relaxing in a sitting position.

The first part of this exercise—stretching the back and arms upwards and lungs full while in a sitting position—strengthens the lungs, and tones the heart and the abdominal organs.

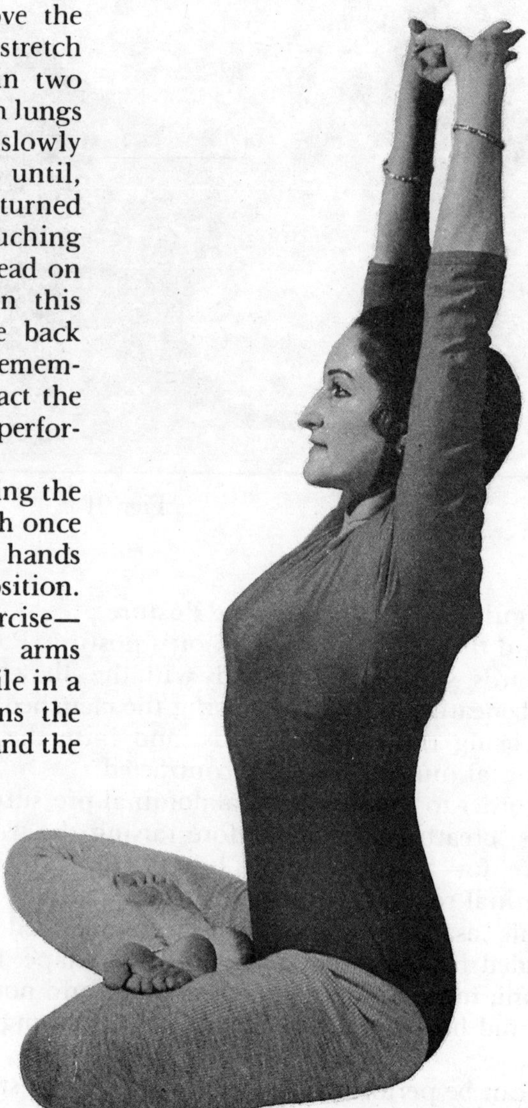

Fig. 92

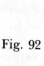

138

The second part—trunk bent forwards and lungs empty—continues the stretching of the spinal column.

Yoga-Mudra fortifies the abdominal muscles, and tones up the uterus and ovaries. The fact that the legs are in the Lotus position with foot lock—heels on either side of the groin—increases intra-abdominal pressure. This exercise is an excellent remedy for the inverted uterus. It is not recommended for those suffering from abdominal problems or high blood pressure. Yoga-Mudra can be practised two or three times in succession.

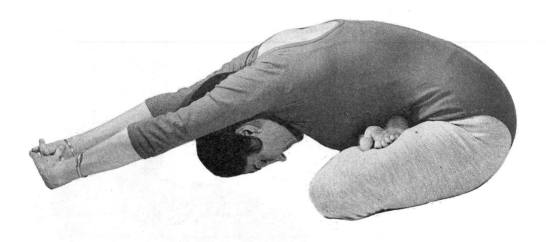

Fig. 93

Shashankasana* : The Hare Posture

The only difference between this exercise and the previous·one is that the legs are in another position. For *Shashankasana*, adopt a kneeling position and sit on the heels. As in Yoga-Mudra, inhale while stretching the trunk and arms upwards, then lean forward while at the same time breathing out. Hold the posture with lungs empty for five seconds while contracting the abdominal muscles and drawing in the abdominal wall. Bring the trunk and arms up again, while breathing in deeply. Stretch once again, lower the arms while breathing out and relax. Direct the attention towards the abdominal region.

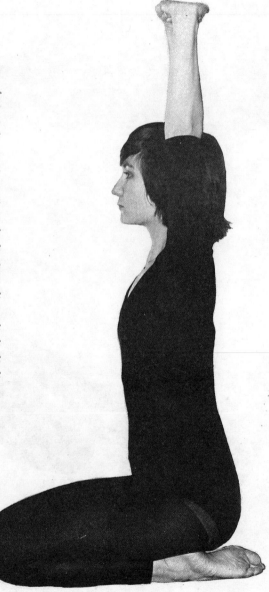

Fig. 94

140

Yoga-Mudra and Shashankasana produce similar beneficial effects, but owing to the different position of the legs, the two exercises do not act on the pelvis and abdominal wall in quite the same way.

The Hare Posture is well-known for its tonic effect on the pelvic region. Like Yoga-Mudra, it remedies uterine inversion. The same restrictions apply to both exercises. Shashankasana can be performed three to five times in succession.

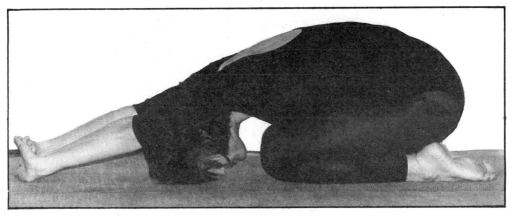

Fig. 95

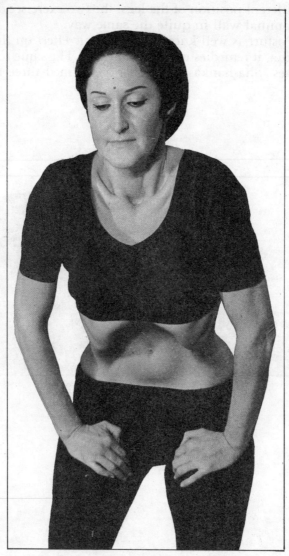

Fig. 96

Uddiyana-Bandha : Raising of the Diaphragm

Adopt a standing position, feet slightly apart. Bend the kness a little, and place the hands on the top of the thighs. Perform one deep inhalation in three parts, and then exhale completely. While keeping the trunk tilted slightly forwards and pushing the hands against the thighs. contract and draw in the abdominal wall, and hollow the stomach by raising the diaphragm and ribs. This upward movement of the diaphragm exerts pressure on the base of the neck, thereby producing visible hollows in the clavicular area.

142

Hold the posture, lungs completely empty, for some five seconds, then breathe in deeply while relaxing the abdominal muscles and bringing the trunk back to an upright position. The exercise can be repeated two to five times. The attention should be directed towards the abdominal region.

Uddiyana-Bandha ensures the correct functioning of the internal organs and fosters control of the abdominal muscles. It is a highly effective way of reducing the volume of the abdomen when distended by pregnancy.

It is not recommended for those suffering from high or low blood pressure, or from abdominal or circulatory problems. Before performing this Bandha, we recommend regular practice of the other exercises described in the present chapter.

Exercises for a Short Session at Home

Young mothers in the throes of breast-feeding and caring for their baby are often heavily occupied with housekeeping. Relaxation and keeping fit are therefore an important need, and mothers should be able to practise the post-natal exercises while remaining at home.

We have composed a short daily session of Hathayoga which permits mothers to perform the following exercises as of the seventh week after childbirth. This presupposes, of course, that the mothers in question are not suffering from health problems.

The exercises should be practised with caution, under the guidance of an expert. The session has been devised for mothers who have followed the Yoga course for pregnant women. A large number of the exercises already learned on the course are repeated here, for they also produce beneficial effects after childbirth. In order to practise them without difficulty, mothers should be thoroughly familiar with them, either by having performed them personally, or by having seen them demonstrated during the course, in the case of certain simple asanas.

There are two exceptions to the asanas recommended for the short home-session, namely Tolangulasana and Yoga-Mudra, which can neither be performed during pregnancy nor learned through a simple demonstration. They are reserved for women who have practised them before becoming pregnant.

Yoga-Mudra can be replaced by Shashankasana, the first part of which is practised regularly throughout the course. The second part—trunk bent forward—is demonstrated by the teacher, but can also be performed during the first stages of pregnancy, knees apart.

Two other exercises—Viparita Karani and Ujjayi Pranayama—are included in the session, but they call for the remarks discussed below.

Those who have not learned to perform Viparita Karani before pregnancy should practise the modified version, as performed during the course for pregnant women, i.e. with the feet against the wall. It is possible, however, to try taking, first, one foot then the other away from the wall, having raised the pelvis and stretched out the legs, in order to adopt the unmodified inverted position.

Whether modified or not, Viparita Karani is highly beneficial to women who are breast-feeding because it stimulates the pituitary gland producing the hornomes required for breast-feeding and the reconstitution of the menstrual cycle. The proper functioning of the pituitary gland is essential to that of the uterus and ovaries.

Fig. 74

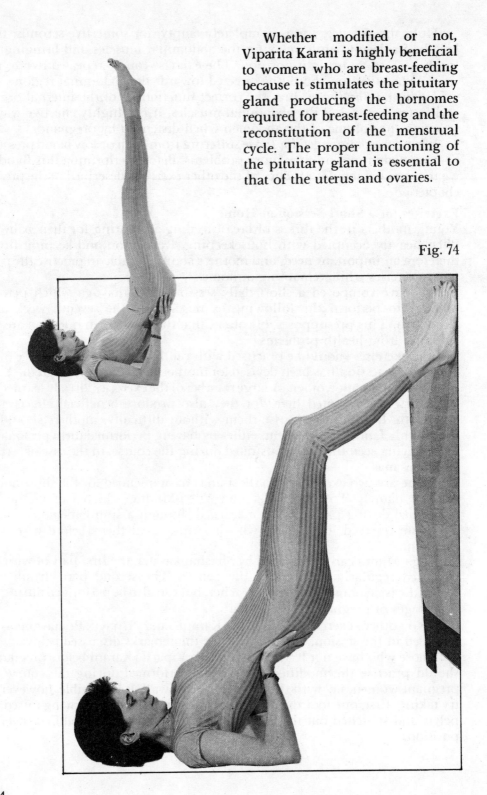

144

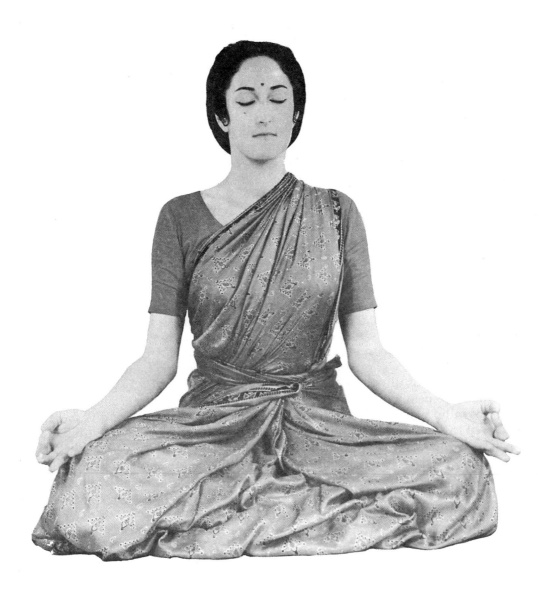

As for Ujjayi Pranayama, it is important to note that a slightly different breathing technique is used after, as opposed to during, pregnancy. In the post-natal version, when exhaling, the contraction of the abdominal muscles is stronger. The mother must gradually draw in the abdominal wall to its fullest extent, a movement which cannot be performed during pregnancy. This increasingly strong contraction should be continued until there is no air left in the lungs.

During inhalation, first, the abdominal wall should be slightly arched by lowering the diaphragm, and then the ribs should be fully expanded. Throughout the duration of the Pranayama, the abdominal muscles must remain under control and should never be allowed to relax completely.

Apart from the highly beneficial effects this exercise produces on the nervous system and the internal organs, it also helps the abdomen distorted by pregnancy to regain its initial shape.

We shall now examine the part of the session devoted to complete Yogic breathing and relaxation, as well as to interiorisation. There is no need to wait six weeks before practising them. Breathing and relaxation can already be performed while the mother is still lying in bed at the hospital. This will help her recuperate more quickly and easily from the exhaustion caused by childbirth. As soon as she returns home, she can also practise interiorisation.

Once the child has arrived, the young mother is faced with a very different kind of family life, especially if it is her first child.

In the West, the mother must often perform household chores completely unassisted. She must not only cope with the fatigue caused by childbirth, the care of her newborn baby, and her lack of experience, but also with the fear that she may not be equal to her new tasks. This explains why young mothers sometimes risk going into depression. Rendered even more sensitive by the hormonal transformation which takes place within the body after childbirth, they come under considerable psychic stress, feel lifeless, despondent, and overwhelmed by events. It is imperative for the young mother to find time for relaxing so that she can eliminate fatigue and nervous tension.

The fact that she has regularly practised Yogic breathing and Savasana, the posture of tranquillity and complete relaxation, during the Yoga course for pregnant women, will now prove to be of very great help indeed. The mother's state of mind plays an important part in helping the milk to rise, and there is no need to emphazise how important the mother's milk is to the health of the newborn child.

Anxiety, irritableness, and heavy physical or moral fatigue prevent the normal process of breast-feeding and do not allow the mother fully to benefit from the joys of having given birth to a child. Interiorisation is the best way of re-establishing contact with oneself, calming the mind, and controlling the emotions.

We recommend practising the exercises described in Chapter 2, "Exercises for Over-coming Emotional Stress." in order to prevent the build-up of emotional tension. The following are exercises for a session lasting roughly half an hour:

1. Stretching the back : Cross-legged (Fig. 24), repeat three times.

2. Complete Yogic Breathing : Cross-legged or in the Half-Lotus position (See p 60), perform five to ten times.

3. Asvini-Mudra* : Symbol of the Mare in the Knee-Chest Posture, repeat two series of three to five contractions (Fig. 50).

4. Ardha-Halasana* : Half-Plough posture. Begin by raising one leg at a time, repeat this exercise two or three times on each side (Fig. 54).

5. Utthitapada-Merudandasana* : Spinal column posture, legs raised (Fig. 88), repeat two to four times for five seconds.

Having practised for a week, one of the following three exercises may be added :

6a. Paripurna-Navasana* : Boat posture (Fig. 89). Or

6b. Variation* : Boat posture, hands on ground (Fig. 90), is easier to perform and which should be used to begin with. Or

6c. Tolangulasana* : Balance posture, (Fig. 91) can only be performed by those who have practised it before becoming pregnant.

The exercise chosen can be repeated two or three times for several seconds.

7. Ustrasana : Camel posture, (Fig. 55) should be practised two or three times from three to five seconds. This exercise can be alternated with Catuspadasana*, i.e. Cat posture (Fig. 62).

8a. Shashankasana* : Hare posture, (Fig. 94) should be performed three to five times for five seconds. Or

8b. Yoga-Mudra, Variation* : With stretching of back and arms, (Fig. 93) can only be performed by those who have already practised it before becoming pregnant. Should be repeated two or three times for five seconds.

9. Viparita Karani : Inverted position. (Fig. 73 & 74). This modified exercise has already been practised during pregnancy and can now be performed with or without the modification. It should be repeated once or twice for fifteen seconds to two minutes. The duration can be increased by five seconds every week if practised daily. This inverted position is not recommended to those with high blood pressure.

10. Savasana : Complete Yogic relaxation, (Fig. 79) should be performed once for five to ten minutes.

11a. Ujjayi Pranayama : Breathing with glottis partly closed, (Fig. 81,) should be repeated five to twelve times. Or

11b. Anuloma Viloma Pranayama : Breathing through alternate nostrills, (Fig. 82),repeat three to seven times.

12. Interiorisation : (Fig. 18).

---

* All asanas marked with an asterisk (*) should not be performed during menstruation.

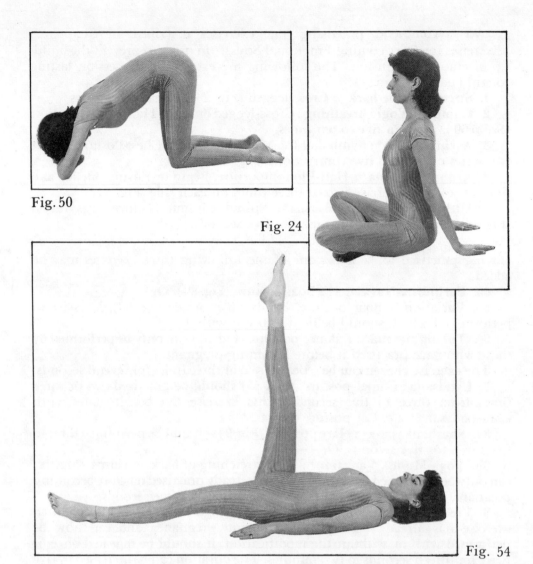

Fig. 50

Fig. 24

Fig. 54

Fig. 88

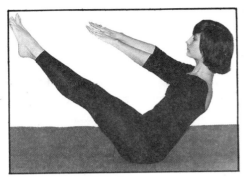

Fig. 89

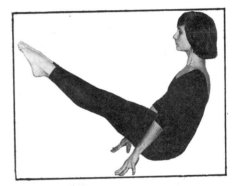

Fig. 91

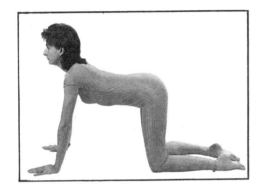

Fig. 62

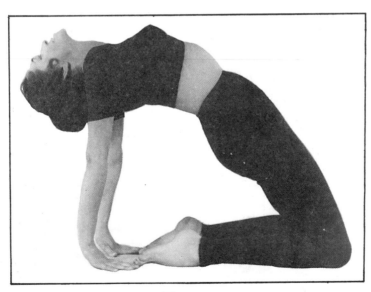

Fig. 90

Fig. 55

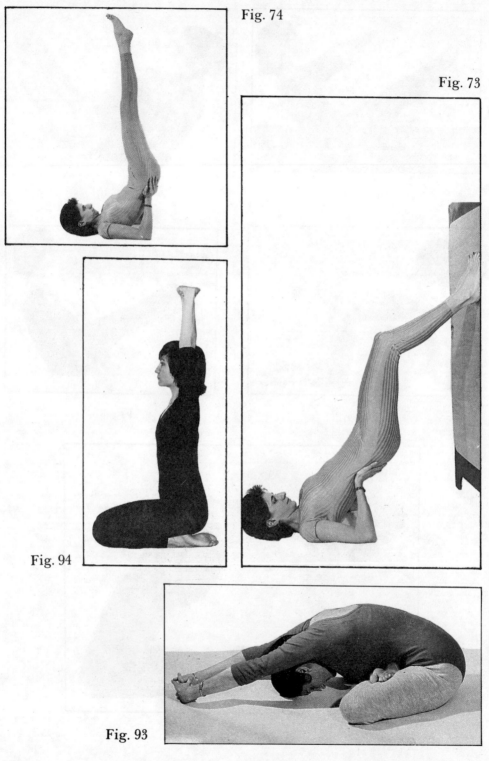

Fig. 74

Fig. 73

Fig. 94

Fig. 93

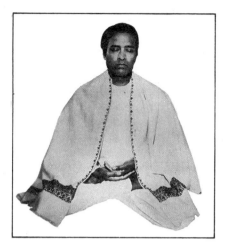

Fig. 18

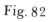

Fig. 82

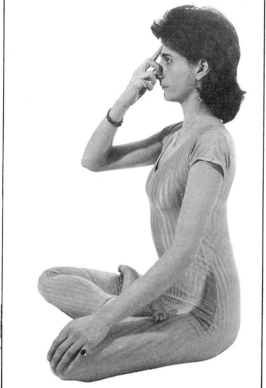

Fig. 81

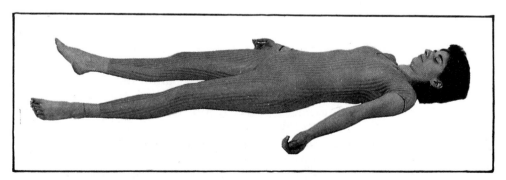

Fig. 79

Wisdom of Yoga

Be with caution bold.

SWAMI KUVALAYANANDA

For Hathayoga to give best results, it must be practised regularly with patience and perseverance. Hathayoga is of great benefit to each and every one of us, but only if it is practised in its entirety, as conceived and elaborated over the centuries by the great Yogis and Rishis of India, and as it continues to be taught by *bona fide* experts of today.

Let us remember that the aim of Yoga is to go beyond our corporal limits and to transcend identification with the physical body in order to attain ever-higher degrees of consciousness.

Many people, however, are only interested in the Yogic postures and practise them for no other reason than to keep physically fit. They make no attempt to purify their mental state, and fail to realize that a confused, uncontrolled mind can produce harmful effects on their physical state.

For a person to be completely fulfilled, his mind must control his body and not the opposite. In Hathayoga, discipline of the body must encourage the mind. It is essential, therefore, to combine the physical exercises of Yoga with interiorisation and meditation. These will increase the individual's knowledge of himself, improve his character, and help him evolve on a spiritual plane. Once one progresses along the path of Yoga, the wish to practise meditation comes quite naturally.

One should begin with interiorisation accompanied by Yogic breathing. Once the nervous system and the mind have been sufficiently prepared and purified by these exercises, as well as by a healthy way of life, meditation will be successful and lead to equanimity, inner peace and bliss.

Pratyahara is an interiorisation exercise during which the sensory organs are no longer directed towards external objects. In the words of Sri Ramakrishna: "By turning the mind within, oneself one acquires discrimination and through discrimination one finds Truth." As for meditation, it is concentration on the Self which resides in the heart of each individual. The Self is the Substance of our soul. It is pure Awareness.

Meditation is an act performed by our soul and consciousness, the aim of which is union with Divine Consciousness. *Like a drop of water which falls into the sea and merges with it, so in meditation the individual consciousness plunges into the Universal Consciousness and becomes one with it.* Thus the complete practice of Hathayogic ensures us not only perfect physical health, but also gives us incalculable moral and spiritual strength, as well as the energy required to overcome obstacles and progress quickly along the path of Life.

May parents who wish to procreate set an example by cultivating their mind in dignity and wisdom. May they be peace-loving and altruistic so that their children are born and grow up in a serene, harmonious atmosphere, and live happily on earth. May the new generation in their turn grow into well-balanced, reliable men and women, so that they may play a worthy part in society and be filled with love for all mankind.

> *All expansion is life.*
> *All contraction is death.*
> *All love is expansion.*
> *All selfishness is contraction.*
> *Love is therefore the only law of life.*

Swami Vivekananda

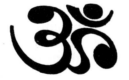

INDIAN FOOD USUALLY TAKES a long time to prepare and is often too spicy for Western tastes. The recipes contained in this chapter include only products which are available in specialized food shops. They have been simplified for faster preparation. None of the dishes described contains strong seasoning or spices, for these are not recommended for pregnant women in any case.

The quantities given serve two.

Two Important Rules

1. Food and drinks should be served neither too hot nor too cold.

2. Vegetables should be fresh and preferably naturally grown. They should be lightly cooked over a low flame in order to preserve all the vitamins they contain.

Herbs and Spices, and their Beneficial Effects on the Health, as Described by *Ayurveda*

a) **Saffron** : Either in stigmas or powder, gives a healthy complexion and skin to the mother and child. It prevents pimples and boils from forming, guards against hiccoughs and feelings of nausea, and is good for the eyes.

b) **Curcuma** : Turmeric or *Haldi* is also beneficial to the complexion, fights flatulence, and is an effective vermicide![1]   It is very good for a troublesome uterus, and being bitter, purifies breast-milk.

c) **Cominos** : *Jeeraka* or Iranian cumin comes in either seed or powder form. It reduces swelling of the uterus, purifies the blood and keeps the complexion healthy, stimulates the digestion, increases breast-milk, acts as a diuretic and kills worms.[2]

d) **Black pepper** : *Kali Mirch* helps fight digestive problems and constipation, acts as a diuretic, and brings relief from chronic colds.

e) **Mustard seeds** : *Sarson* stimulates the appetite and are used to fight throat diseases.

---

1. Introduction to Ayurveda, Dr. C.G. Thakkur.
2. Ibid.

f) Coriander : *Dhania,* either seeds or powder, is good for the health in general. Fresh coriander leaves remove heartburn, and acts as an appetizer and a digestive.

g) Cinnamon : *Dalchini* purifies the throat. fights coughs, and sinus troubles and worms.

h) Cardamom : *Ilaichi* which comes in either seed or powder form, has a tonic and diuretic effect, is good for the heat, calms heartburn, and remedies coughs.

i) Cloves : *Laung* are used against coughs, asthma and hiccoughs. They also purify the blood.

j) Tamarind : *Imli* usually available dried, is good for the heart, liver and kidneys. Although it stimulates the appetite and digestion, if taken in too large a quantity, tamarind provokes dyspepsia.

Recipes

Rice

Basmati (also available in the West) is a particularly good Indian rice, and can be used in the following preparation of the plain, Indian-style rice which accompanies many dishes. First remove any impurities from the *Basmati* rice. Wash several times, then leave to soak for one hour. Rinse and pour into a saucepan of either salted or unsalted boiling water; two parts of water to one part of rice. Bring to the boil again, then lower the flame. Cover and cook for eight minutes. Rice must always be properly cooked to avoid gastric problems. Cooking time varies considerably, according to the quality of the rice.

Almond (or Cashew) and Raisin Pullao
   3 bowls of cooked rice
   3 cardamom seeds, peeled and crushed
   3 grains of pepper, crushed
   3 cloves, crushed
   1 stick of cinnamon, 1 cm, divided into small sections, or 3 pinches of each of these spices if in powder form 1 onion (optional)
   1 handful of raisins
   1 handful of halved almonds or cashew nuts
   1 soupspoon of oil or butter
   salt

Heat the oil or butter in a frying pan. Fry onions till they turn brown. Then add the almonds or cashew nuts, spices and raisins. Allow to fry for a few moments. As soon as the almonds are browned, add the three bowls of rice, salt to taste. Stir all the ingredients together, then allow to cook for two or three minutes. Serve.

Lemon Rice
   3 bowls of cooked rice
   1/4 teaspoon of powdered curcuma (turmeric)
   1/2 teaspoon of mustard seeds
   1 soupspoon of either fresh or dessicated grated coconut 3 or 4 leaves of fresh or dried curry leaves (or one or two bay leaves cut into strips)

155

1 handful of salted peanuts (or cashew nuts), cut into halves. Juice of one
lemon
salt
1 soupspoon of oil

Heat one soupspoon of oil in a frying pan. Drop the mustard seeds into the
pan and allow to burst i.e. Chhauk on a low flame, taking care to cover the
pan. Add the curcuma and brown with the curry or bay leaves (*Tej Patta*). Add
the rice, the soupspoon of coconut, the lemon juice and the peanuts or cashew
nuts. Stir thoroughly, cover the pan, and allow to cook for two to three
minutes. Serve.

Saffron Rice
This is obtained by adding three pinches or 1/4 teaspoon of saffron to the
water used to boil the rice.

Dhal : a kind of lentil
Dhal is served either with rice or with wholewheat cakes known as *chapatis*.
Indian families eat dhal at least once a day, for it is one of the most protein-rich
and least costly foods.

In Europe, two kinds of dhal are obtainable : *masur* (small pinkish-orange
lentils) and *chana* (yellow lentils resembling split green peas).

Although we have given recipes for *masur* and *chana*, other kinds of white
or green lentils, split peas or chick peas can be prepared in the same way.

Masur Dhal with Tomatoes
1 teacup masur dhal
2 halved tomatoes
1 small lump of dried tamarind, soaked in a cup of hot water for several
minutes, then squeezed out
(or juice of 1/2 lemon instead)
4 or 5 fresh or dried curry leaves
1/4 teaspoon mustard seeds
1 chopped onion (optional)
1/4 teaspoon powdered curcuma
1 small teaspoon powdered cominos
1 small teaspoon powdered coriander
1 soupspoon grated coconut
1 soupspoon ground-nut oil
salt

Remove impurities from the dhal and wash. Allow to soak in luke warm
water for half an hour. Rinse. Cook in five cups of cold water on a high flame
for five minutes, making to skim off the froth. Lower the flame and allow the
dhal to simmer until soft and tender. Strain the tamarind and pour on a little
more water as it is added to the dhal (if tamarind is not available, lemon juice
may be used). Add the spices, salt, onion, tomatoes, coconut and curry leave
(*Kadi Patta*), and allow to cook. Burst (i.e. *Chhauk*) the mustard seeds in a
small, covered frying pan, without burning them, and immediately pour them
onto the dhal as it is cooking.

Masur dhal usually requires 15 minutes cooking time, but it can sometimes take up to one hour or more, depending on the quality of the lentils. When ready, it should have the consistency of a fairly liquid soup. If necessary, water may be added during cooking. Masur dhal is served with plain rice and curd.

Chana Dhal with Celery

1 rounded teacup of chana dhal
2 sticks of celery (i.e. *Agwan*), chopped into pieces 4 cm long
1 tomato, halved
1 soupspoon oil
salt
Spices and quantities same as for masur dhal
1 small lump (1.5 cm diameter) of tamarind or juice of half a lemon)
1/4 teaspoon curcuma
1 small teaspoon cominos
1 small teaspoon coriander
1 soupspoon grated coconut
3 or 4 curry leaves
1/4 teaspoon mustard seeds

Remove impurities from the dhal and wash. Allow to soak for 1/2 hour in luke warm water. Rinse. Cook in eight cups of cold water. Bring to the boil and skim. Cook for ten minutes, then lower the flame. Simmer until soft and tender. Add the tamarind (see masur dhal) or lemon juice, spices, celery coconut and tomato. Continue to simmer, adding water if necessary, until the celery is completely cooked. Add salt when vegetables are almost tender. Burst the mustard seeds as for the masur dhal and add to the chana dhal before removing from flame. When ready, the chana dhal should have a soup-like consistency. Serve with rice and curd.

Variation 1 : The celery sticks can be replaced by green beans, a leek or small courgette such as marrow of banana stem, drum sticks etc, or a small aubergine chopped such as fruits of egg-plants or like the celery. It is also possible to mix several vegetables, e.g. a carrot, turnip, tomato and onion.

Variation 2 : The dhal and vegetables can be cooked using no other spices but curcuma, mustard seeds and tamarind (or lemon juice).

Variation 3 : Add to plain dhal (i.e. without spices) one onion, chopped and well browned in oil or butter, and chopped fresh coriander leaves, just before serving.

Green Soya Beans with Courgettes

Green soya beans can be cooked in the same way as the dhal.

1 cup soya beans
1 tomato, halved
1 courgette, cut into slices 4 cm long
1 small chopped onion (optional)
salt
Spices same as for the two types of dhal already described :
1 small lump tamarind (or juice of 1/2 lemon)
1/4 teaspoon curcuma

1 small teaspoon cominos
1 small teaspoon coriander
1/4 teaspoon mustard seed

Bhajis Indian-Style Vegetables

In India, the word 'curry' is used to designate a spicy sauce in which vegetables, fish, chicken or mutton is cooked.

Mutter Curry with Mushrooms (peas with mushrooms)

200 g freshly shelled peas
12 fresh cultivated mushrooms
1 peeled chopped tomato
1 large onion, finely chopped
1 or 2 cloves of garlic, crushed
salt
2 or 3 soupspoon of butter or oil
3/4 teaspoon powdered curcuma
3/4 teaspoon garam masala, i.e. :
3 peeled, crushed cardamoms
3 crushed cloves
3 ground pepper seeds
3 pinches of cinnamon, all of which is mixed together

To clean the mushrooms, wash, brush or peel them, and cut them into slices. Brown the onion in the oil or butter. Add the peeled chopped tomato, crushed garlic, the curcuma and the *garam masala*. Mix together. Add the peas and mushroom, and stir fry for five minutes. Pour in two glasses of water, cover and allow to simmer until the vegetables are tender (roughly 20 minutes). If the liquid reduces, add more water to make a sauce. Salt when almost cooked, and serve with plain rice.

Baingan Curry (Aubergine curry)

1 small unpeeled aubergine, sliced
1 peeled chopped tomato
1 small sweet pepper (capsicum), diced
1 chopped onion
1 or 2 cloves of garlic, crushed
1/2 teaspoon of mustard seeds
1 small lump of fresh or dried tamarind
several curry leaves
1 soupspoon Madras curry powder
2 soupspoons ground-nut oil
salt
Fresh chopped coriander leaves (optional)

Heat the oil, then lower the flame. Burst the mustard seeds, making sure to cover the saucepan. Add the onion and brown, then add the curry leaves and tomato. Allow to cook for several minutes, then pour in the seived tamarind juice (See Masur Dhal) and two or three glasses of water. Bring to the boil and add the curry powder, garlic, sweet pepper (capsicum) and aubergine. When almost cooked add salt. The dish can be sprinkled with coriander leaves, chopped like parsley, and seasoned with grated garlic. Serve with plain rice.

Desserts

Gajer ka Halwa (Carrot Halva)

400 g carrots

1/2 litre milk

100 g unrefined sugar

1 handful crushed cashew nuts or almonds

1/2 teaspoon powdered cardamom

1 soupspoon butter

Wash, peel, and finely grate the carrots. Cook for roughly 3/4 hour in the milk on a low flame until soft and tender, stirring from time to time. Add the sugar and stir until quite solid. Add the butter, nuts and cardamom, and continue cooking until all the liquid has been absorbed. Serve warm.

Nariel Barfi : Coconut Cakes

1 finely grated coconut (brown part removed)

1/4 litre milk

450 g unrefined brown sugar

1/2 soupspoons orange flower water

1 soupspoon butter (to grease dish)

Dissolve the sugar in the milk in a frying pan over a low flame. Add the coconut and cook, stirring until the mixture become solid. When nearly cooked, add a knob of butter. Remove from flame and pour on the orange flower water and mix. Transfer to a small greased caketin. The cake should be roughly 2 cm thick. Allow to cool, then cut into rectangles. Serves 4 to 6.

Dessicated coconut cooks more quickly (roughly in 10 minutes), and if it is used, we recommend the following recipe. Serves 2 or 3.

125 g dessicated coconut

1.5 decilitres milk

200 g unrefined sugar

1 1/2 soupspoon orange flower water small quantity of butter

Dr. Bircher's Müesli : Swiss speciality

Soak six rounded soupspoons of oats in 200 ml fresh milk. Add three soupspoons of unrefined brown sugar (according to taste), one soupspoon grated almonds, the juice of one lemon, and one grated apple.

According to taste, it is also possible to add a chopped or mashed banana, fresh grapes, a diced orange or pear, etc., as well as dried fruits : figs, raisins, apricots, walnuts, dates, prunes, etc. To give more flavour to the müesli, one can add sweetened pure condensed milk or decorate it with whipped cream serves two.

Variation : When strawberries are in season, it is possible to prepare the müesli with them, either chopped or pureed, adding a banana. Whatever the variation, lemon juice should be added. The fresh milk can also be replaced with condensed milk diluted in a small amount of water, or one or two pots of curd.

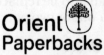